STRONG

GIACOMO FARCI

FOREWORD BY MARK STRONG

ISBN 978-1-9161041-0-5

For my wife,
who inspires me every day.

For my brother,
who showed me how to walk without fear.

For my parents,
who made the pillars of my temple.

CONTENTS

FOREWORD BY MARK STRONG

I'm over 50 and in the best shape of my life — not only physically, but also mentally. Most of the time I try to eat, train and rest in a way that sustains my energy levels and allows me to engage with, be present for, and enjoy my work, family and friends.

This wasn't always the case — for years I wasn't as fit as I wish I could have been, despite many fitness and nutritional plans, which I tried to stick to. I always liked a good sweat, but sometimes just the thought of going to the gym or for a run felt like an unbearable chore. Other times, I would succumb to a meal full of sugar even though there were better options, and that was annoying. Although I've always been very driven in my professional life, for reasons I couldn't quite understand, maintaining the motivation to stick to fitness and nutrition plans was difficult. I'd try harder, put in more effort and use more willpower — but somehow it didn't work, and when it did work, it didn't last. Instead, I often found myself demotivated and not in the frame of mind to go for a run, and I'd end up eating or drinking something unhealthy. I used to resent my lifestyle and busy schedule for lack of results, and would feel somehow stuck.

At 47, a producer introduced me to Giacomo Farci to prepare for an action film where I had to not only look good but also be fit enough to climb walls, fight and run. I was told that Giac was 'not your normal personal trainer' and I was nervous knowing he was a former Italian national kickboxing champion. I expected hard-core training, strict dieting, and shouted motivational quotes like his predecessors used to do. Instead, at our first meeting seated at a table, he asked about my daily and weekly schedules, what my work dynamics were, my family life and, interestingly, my reaction to social situations where drinking and eating a certain way was expected. I quickly understood Giac wasn't just in the business of selling protein shakes.

We talked about how feelings might have an effect on cravings for sugar and about the quality of sleep and energy levels through the day. I was surprised to hear that the correct technique for squats, deadlifts, bench press and chin-ups is not rocket science, and that a good trainer can train you to execute them properly after a bit of practice. Same with nutrition — most systems (like intermittent fasting or diets) all work for an objective but how do you make yourself able to get ready, commute to the gym and exercise with mindfulness when certain specific factors peculiar to your lifestyle get in the way? How do you resist food cravings and avoid drinking at social events that are built around drinking? Those were my questions among many others.

After working with Giac, I got into excellent shape for the film and enjoyed the process so much that after many years of working with him, I still manage to stay in great shape without too much effort by using the right strategies. I manage to keep off the unwanted body fat while maintaining muscle mass. My health is better and I don't get those annoying colds anymore. The quality of my sleep could improve but thanks to Giac I am working on it.

Friends and colleagues have asked me how I manage to do it *despite* my lifestyle with its busy schedule, but the reality is that I want to be fit in mind and body to *support* my lifestyle. The way I eat, train and rest is the way i support my work and social life. That's where the idea for this book came from — We felt it would be useful for Giac to write what he does on a daily basis with his clients and share it.

Read on to see which strategies and tools you can use to keep as close as possible to your aesthetic, fitness, health, career and family goals.

It really can start here.

Mark Strong

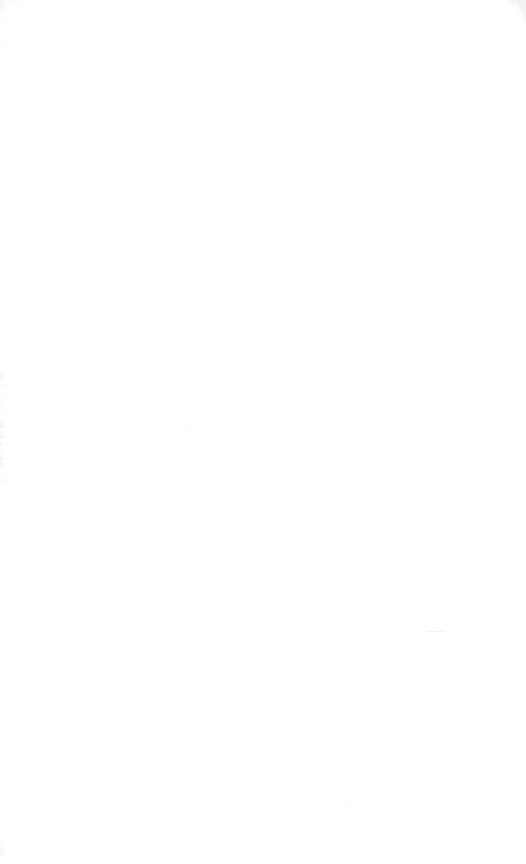

INTRODUCTION

The aim of this book is to help you improve your daily diet and keep consistency with your fitness schedule, while using less (and not wasting any) precious resources like time and will-power, and without compromising your busy lifestyle. If you will implement even only one new strategy per chapter in your daily life, step by step, you will notice a big positive change.

Make no mistake, this is not another book about the best diet and the best exercise regime. There is already lot of informative material and tools out there: great books and smart phone fitness apps, fitness TV channels and websites, great gyms and sport centres, qualified personal trainers and nutritionists.

In fact, we should all know how to eat and work out yet still, sometimes, it feels so hard to do. How can we reduce the chances of overeating and drinking too much? How can we make sure that our precious available time to work out doesn't go wasted due to a decline in motivation and inspiration? The aim of this book is to help you get the most from your daily diet and to help you keep consistency with your fitness schedule.

To be clear, with the word 'diet' I refer to the original meaning from the ancient Greek *diaita*, which means 'way of living'. Whatever you are eating is your diet, which can be more or less rigid. You might count calories, and/or keep 'macros' (protein, carbohydrates, fat) and 'micros' (vitamins, minerals) in check, or you might only use general guidelines like avoiding processed foods, refined sugar, etc. Whatever you are eating is your diet, and your diet ultimately determines the way you feel and function while supporting your lifestyle and health.

By fitness schedule I mean every workout at the gym (resistance training, spinning, etc.) or every sports match with your friends (football, tennis, golf, etc.) or every physical activity (rock climbing, swimming, cycling, etc.). In a few words, everything that requires a decent level of physical effort that is booked into your calendar and you don't want to miss.

Now let me share with you these tools and strategies, along with stories of how my clients incorporated them into their lives to achieve their success.

Let's start.

Giac Farci

1

MIND SPACE

Precisely like a computer that runs its programs over an allocated memory space, our brain runs its analytic and problem-solving processes over a network of physical structures that for simplicity I'll refer to here as *mind space*.

- **The amount of mind space that you keep free and available during a busy day will ultimately determine your capacity to stay on top of your diet and fitness schedule**

When I analyse more than a decade of data that I collected in my diary, I see the most frequent reasons given by my clients for cancelling their sessions with me were:

34% – Last minute **work issues.**
Most common reasons were 'I'm stuck in a meeting' or 'I have a last-minute work issue'.

30% – Overcrowded **mind space.**

A few examples of texts and emails:

▶ Session booked for 12.30pm. Text at 11.30am: 'Sorry Giac, I cannot make it today, work is very busy, and I am not in the right frame of mind for training. Apologies.'

▶ Session booked for 7pm. Text at 6.30pm: 'Giac, I had a really bad day, I'm going home. Sorry but I don't have my head in the right place.'

26% – Feeling run-down due to **poor sleep**.

7% – Having a **hangover**. Most of the time caused by a work/social event.

3% – Other. For example: a family crisis like an unplanned pick-up for kids from school; parents' or grandparents' poor health; transport disruptions).

It is clear that, apart from not having enough time, having an overcrowded mind space is major obstacle to maintaining a consistent fitness program.

● An overcrowded mind space can make your precious available time worthless.

Very often, the next time that I see those clients who cancelled their sessions due to overcrowded mind space, when I ask whether they had at least eaten as they should do (according to the plan), the most common response is: 'No, I haven't done it. I could, but I haven't. I don't know why. Instead, I had pasta/pizza/crisps.'

The amount of mind space available during the day will determine the level of their creativity and inspiration, their capacity to connect with the people who matter, and their consistency with their fitness schedule and diet.

The reason we need mind space

Many modern jobs require mental productivity over physical effort. Jobs, family, and social life combined require our brains to handle a lot: solving problems, handling crises, choosing priorities, recognising opportunities, generating new ideas, staying inspired, successfully communicating with co-workers, clients and dear ones.

To effectively manage these processes, we need sufficient available mind space. When we have it, every problem has a solution, every goal seems achievable, our relationships work, we feel in control and motivated.

No matter how powerful a computer is, when it runs too many programs at the same time, it reaches capacity — and the human brain is exactly the same. When capacity is reached, the whole system starts to slow down and lose performance. If a computer fails to shut down a few programs, the entire system gets slower exponentially and ultimately freezes. It therefore needs to be re-booted.

In the same way, when our mind space gets overcrowded, our processes slow down. Every problem takes longer to solve. For example, you could be working for many hours trying to find a solution to a problem on a business deal, a project, a script or a song, without success. If we're feeling overwhelmed and overburdened, at some point we start feeling disengaged with our projects, totally uninspired and not creative. But if we take a break and go for a walk, often the solution to the problem appears in your mind. A new inspiring idea that seemingly came from nowhere!

That idea has been generated in the mind space that we managed to free up during that relaxing walk in a stimulating new scenario. We then feel in control again, fully present in the moment, engaged with the project again. We go back to work inspired. But life is not always that simple.

When life is just too much to handle with unforeseen work issues and family crises, on top of an already hectic schedule, it's easy to feel overwhelmed and unable to focus, resulting in us losing analytic capacity and struggling to prioritise. We stall and we think that there is not enough time to accomplish all the important things. We believe that our lives are too hectic and we don't have control over it. Yet, in the desperate and vain attempt to get back in control, we make very strange decisions that go against our master plan, decisions that lead to the wasting of our precious time. It usually happens in two ways: procrastination or craving comfort food and drinks.

Reaction 1: Procrastination

Procrastination is avoiding what we know we should be doing. Instead, we do something else that isn't important. We decide to do a task that isn't immediately necessary or a priority, instead of the more important job.

As a result of procrastination, we waste our precious available time. We miss opportunities. We don't get any closer to our goals, and actually sometimes we fall even further behind. Say you have a scheduled lunchtime run in your diary but instead *choose* to delay that run to check funny/sports videos on a social network, or read the latest spoilers of your favourite TV series. You plan to do it *only for 2 minutes*, then realise 30 minutes later that the only available time in the day for that run is now gone.

Or, after a difficult day at work, instead of hitting the gym as planned, you decide to go home because you 'need to unwind'. We then regret that decision almost immediately after sitting down on the sofa. We feel surprised and annoyed with our lack of discipline. In both situations, we planned to get back in control of life, procrastinated and felt even more out of control afterwards.

Procrastination is more likely to affect our fitness routine rather than work or family schedule because we all have a boss to report to, and loved ones who depend on us. However, with fitness, we are entirely in charge but also left alone. You are your own captain, and therefore it becomes much harder to manage when working out feels like compulsory (and unpaid) work instead of voluntary fun.

When we are overwhelmed and want to *get back in control*, we are more likely to cancel a training session to gain time for ourselves instead of rescheduling a work meeting or missing a family or social event.

The fitness schedule is often the first to be de-prioritized compared to work or family schedules.

17

Reaction 2: Craving comfort food & drinks

If we feel like we've had a tough and overwhelming week, we often decide to 'reward' ourselves with comfort food, a so-called treat which is often a meal with plenty of added sugar, refined flours and trans-fats.

For example, it's 3pm, and we are seated doing a tedious and repetitive task, and so we feel we need a break and something to eat. Even though there is an apple and some nuts available, we decide to go to the closest café and have a sugary pastry. We tell ourselves 'I'm having a bad day, I deserve a treat', and only a moment later, we feel regret and disappointment because we didn't stick to the original diet plan.

Sometimes, even though we planned to go home, eat a healthy dinner early in the evening and have a dry day, we find ourselves in the company of colleagues, making food and drink choices that we will regret in the morning.

These two reactions begin during those moments when the only thing we want to do is pause and take a break from everything, while reaching for some form of reward. Those moments are the ones we need to avoid to keep consistency with a fitness schedule and diet.

The amount of mind space that we manage to keep free and available during a busy day will ultimately determine our capacity to stay on top of our workouts and healthy meals. When our mind space is overcrowded with too much stuff that shouldn't be there, we feel overwhelmed and thinking straight becomes incredibly hard.

We struggle to find a solution to little problems, and every task feels like a chore. We don't feel creative or inspired, we strive to be present in the moment. The desire, motivation, enjoyment and inspiration for doing anything physical fades away and we often look for immediate gratification in the form of sweet treats and sugary snacks._

When we feel overwhelmed, the last thing we want to do is start warming up, stretching, sweating. We avoid working out, or we start a workout and keep shaking our head thinking, *I should be doing something else, I don't want to work out.*

When we feel overburdened, just thinking about putting a few ingredients together to cook or selecting the best food option when on-the-go, feels like an unbearable chore. We are more likely to reach for sugary comfort food to get that instant gratification given by the blood sugar rush.

● **During those overwhelming moments we are more likely to de-prioritize our fitness program and compromise our diet.**

Some say that it works the opposite for them. When they are stressed, they go for a workout and feel better. We surely can go for a long run when we are bored, we can lift weights while angry, we can punch the boxing bag hard when we are frustrated, and we might feel better afterwards. But we are unlikely to do it when we are overwhelmed. During those moments, we normally shake our head and think '*I'm too busy for this, I shouldn't be here.*' That's not a nice place to be.

● ● ●

How to free up your mind space

STRONG is written with 20+ years of experience consulting with highly skilled, high-performing and busy individuals, each of them at the top of their game. I have learnt from every single client, both at the gym after over 20,000 personal training sessions, and outside the gym when spending time with them and their families. I've noticed that although my clients perform in different business and creative fields, they share common tools and strategies to keep mind space available during the day. They are masters of planning, prioritization and juggling between daily tasks and crises, and they use specific tactics to keep available mind space to avoid getting overwhelmed.

1) Keep the internal mind-space de-cluttered

Judy, 41, Managing Director, believes that *your mind shouldn't be your office, neither your diary nor your calendar.*

Things to remember such as to-do lists, bills to pay, dates or hotel ideas for the family trip and business development ideas are like Post-it notes on the office board. Every Post-it occupies space.

How would we feel looking at a board overfilled with Post-its about every little thing? It's confusing. The more clutter in Judy's mind space, the greater the chance of forgetting important things, missing deadlines and opportunities. The brain knows that there is a lot to remember and the risk of omission is high — so it never relaxes.

Judy's system aims to put away every 'to-do', every task, every idea, out of her mind. She puts them into a place where she can store it, record it and visualize it. She uses urgent **to-do lists, short-term project lists, long-term project lists**. Keeping these lists out of her mind gives her more control, by knowing that she can use those lists to retrieve the information when she is ready to tackle each individual task. Judy won't have to worry about it because she is able to access each list when she needs it. She doesn't keep every program open all the time. Judy's system is shared among busy individuals who maintain a high level of productivity in their day.

Another crucial system that these top performers, like Antonie, 44, CEO, use is their **electronic calendar** for all their appointments, work events, social events, business travel, holidays and fitness sessions. In his calendar there are two weekly sessions with me, on the same weekdays at the same time, booked for the year. In this way, Antonie avoids conflicts between events, and effectively plans his fitness schedule and the relaxation time for himself and his family.

His two key mantras are: *if you don't manage your agenda, someone else will,* and *what is not in the diary is not happening.* Top performers like Antonie tend to book all their workouts in their diary at least a full week in advance. This method increases clarity about the upcoming week's fitness routine, and results in a feeling of control and increased motivation to stick to a diet. That's how he manages to keep fit despite a hectic lifestyle.

Another strategy that Judy and Antonie aim to create is electronic-free time for themselves during the day. For example, in order to **keep electronic distractions to a minimum,** they leave their phones in the gym locker to encourage a more mindful approach to working out.

2) Keep the outer space de-cluttered

Lee, 38, film producer, believes that *keeping a tidy and organised environment around him is key to keep a sharper and clearer mind.*

When his environment is cluttered, messy and distracting, his mind starts to be cluttered, messy and distracted. When everything around him is well-organized, functional, creative and inspiring, then he's more likely to feel the same. Clutter bombards our mind with excessive stimuli, which forces our brain to work overtime as more unnecessary programs are running.

Clutter also signals to our brain that there's something else that needs to be done, which is mentally exhausting. There is a deep connection between the space around us and the way we think and feel. If our work desk is messy, it is energy consuming and not enjoyable to keep properly focused on the screen monitor or canvas in front of us. It's exhausting to prepare a meal in a disorganised kitchen, and uninspiring to work out efficiently in a cluttered gym.

Furthermore, a cluttered environment is more likely to slow us down and make us waste time getting things done. Clutter takes up valuable mind space, increasing the chance of feeling overwhelmed, dull and uninspired.

It is not surprising the Royal Marines, very driven and

motivated individuals, say that *a tidy closet makes a tidy mind.* Lee applies this concept not only at work to keep the film set tidy and organised, but to the whole of the environment that surrounds him. His kitchen is free of tempting unhealthy foods, while the surfaces, cupboards and drawers are organised in a way that makes cooking breakfast early in the morning and dinner late at night easy tasks.

Busy individuals like Lee try to keep the environment that they spend time in tidy and functional, be it their office, their home, their garage or their car. What I've come to realise is that there is a correlation between being fit and having a clutter-free environment. Perhaps it is not a coincidence.

● ● ●

This is what the best performers in their fields do to keep mind space available, because they know it is critical to get everything important done during busy days, including maintaining their fitness and diet plan. Sometimes the demands of life make the days hectic. Unforeseen crises and last-minute problems challenge our capacity to prioritize with efficiency. During those moments, mind space becomes overcrowded, increasing the chance for procrastination to kick-in, for the fitness schedule to be de-prioritized, and for a correct diet to be disrupted by reaching for comfort foods.

That's when your capacity to keep strong is disrupted, and the risk of faltering and losing momentum for days — if not weeks — is very high. Below are some strategies to help you keep your consistency with fitness and diet, without compromising your busy lifestyle.

STRONG STRATEGIES

Keep your mind de-cluttered.

▶ **Use short-term and long-term to-do lists.** Put all the info, projects and deadlines somewhere where you can access them whenever you need to.

▶ **Keep a morning journal.** Every morning write 15 lines of whatever ideas, thoughts and feelings you have, without any purpose other than to free your mind. A morning journal is a great tool to free up cognitive resources for other mental activities, including the ability to manage stress more effectively.

▶ **Avoid multitasking.** While constant juggling between a few tasks is the norm in modern life, heavy multitasking creates additional clutter, lowers efficiency, limits attention span and increases stress. The solution is to single-task as much as possible. Make a list of things you need to accomplish that day, keeping the list realistic and straightforward. Start with what's most important and make your way down the list, completing one task at a time, including your training session and meals.

▶ **Take 'white time' to unwind from technology**. The brain needs to rest and recharge to perform smoothly. Set a limit on the amount of time you spend to check your email and social media. Switch off your phone and laptop and do something that makes you feel well, whether it's a long nap, running, or a walk in the park.

Make the environment work for you, not against you.

▶ **Toss and re-organize.** Get rid of all the non-essential items from your work desk, kitchen, studio and garage. Assign a proper place to put everything else.

▶ **Eliminate unhealthy food.** Keep your desk, kitchen shelves, cupboards and draws free of all those foods that you are trying to avoid.

Be in control of your diary.

▶ **Book your workouts in your diary a week in advance.** This increases clarity about what is going to happen fitness-wise in the next few days, and it also gives a feeling of *momentum* which is vital to keep up the motivation to follow a correct diet.

▶ **Do what you enjoy**. Make your fitness schedule enjoyable by booking your favorite class, or book sessions with an inspiring personal trainer and/or training partner to make you

25

more accountable. This will reduce the stress from the anticipation of the workout that is likely to hit when you feel mentally or physically tired.

▶ **Work out where you feel inspired.** Sometimes you only need a change of scene. Many clients over the years have mentioned that they struggled to work out at the gym in the same building where they worked, or close buy. This is because they feel like they never 'leave work' due to proximity and often due to many colleagues being around. I work at studios/gyms and sometimes I struggle to train where I sometimes stay up to 12–14 hours a day. Like many trainers, I work out at different places instead of at the gym where I work, and this is an efficient way to keep motivation high.

▶ **Do what your mind needs**. Different type of sports/training routines have a different effect on different people. Personally, whenever I need to shut my inner dialogue up and go into a state of mindfulness, then I do non-repetitive sports like martial arts (either bag work, pad work or sparring), or wall climbing. They all require a mental break from work and life dynamics in order to solely focus on what I am doing. On the contrary, when I need to let my mind wild and unchained (which is often the source of new valuable ideas) then I choose to do an activity made of repetitive movements like running, swimming or cycling, which don't require too much attention. This is very subjective, therefore you need to find what works for you.

▶ **Use the golden hours.** Whenever possible, get it done in the first available hours of the day. Apart from the great feelings triggered by endorphins, dopamine and other hormones released during and after the workout, there is also a priceless sense of achievement. When you know that you have already completed an essential daily task, you won't think about it anymore, therefore reducing thoughts about working out that occupy mind space. The concept here is that whatever happens during your hectic day, you have already worked out.

▶ **Have a training routine for every situation and environment.** Have a selection of workouts prepared of various lengths to do at the gym, at home, in the park, in a hotel room. This way you can select a workout and go training according to the time you have (60 minutes, 40, 20, even only 10), the available equipment and environment that you are in. Knowing what to do is time effective, motivating and it doesn't take up mental space. Wondering what to do while standing in a crowded gym can be very stressful, demotivating and takes up mind space. Having a written training plan makes it easier to adapt with a few changes in case the gym (or the training location) is too busy.

▶ **When everything feels overwhelming, keep the threshold of your next workout low.** When too much is going on and even the thought of working out feels like an unbearable task, trick your mind by thinking of doing just 5 minutes of stretching. Most of the time, doing just a bit of stretching make you feel somehow activated and keen to carry on with a few more exercises, and sometimes even with a whole session.

2
ROUTINE

High performers streamline their lives in every single aspect and detail. Those who are the best at what they do are efficient and effective by employing faster and simpler methods. I've witnessed how they reduce the amount of time, mental and physical energy necessary for repetitive decisions during the day.

● **Routines reduce decision fatigue while optimising time, preserving willpower and keeping you consistent with your fitness and diet.**

We have a finite amount of willpower for each day. Willpower that is depleted by every decision — big or small — that we have to make. In our crazy, hectic modern life, we're inundated with choices. Should I check email or work on this memo? Should I have lunch at the canteen or somewhere new around the block? Should I lift weights or run today? And so on. Willpower is like a muscle that fatigues during the day, and by the end of the day, our reserve is running on empty.

When this happens, we are mentally tired, irritable and inclined to make poor decisions. When given choices that matter like going to the gym or going home to relax, we'll more likely choose to go home. And after dinner, what about writing our important work memo or watching some TV? Watching TV often wins.

That's why relying on routines over willpower is key especially with those tasks like working out or eating that are repetitive.

The reason you need a routine

The brain is very conservative in terms of energy and tries to do familiar actions.

Think about the last few weekday mornings, what do you actually remember? Probably nothing, as most early mornings blur into one, and recalling one in particular is difficult. You probably don't remember every time you have opened your drawers to pick underwear and socks as it's part of an automatic series of actions that you have done while thinking about something else.

But if your partner decided to swap the content of your drawers, putting the socks in the underwear drawer and vice-versa, then I bet you would remember. You would have a 'freeze', staring at the unexpected content of the familiar drawer for a few seconds while shaking your head in disbelief. Such a small change, such a big disruptor to your day.

What about your last few commutes to work? Difficult to recall all of them, although while on these journeys, you have swerved and moved around many obstacles, hazards and corners. If you were walking, you adapted to different gradients and types of surfaces, slaloming between many people, while alternating the contraction of about 640 skeletal muscles. In the meantime, you probably read the news, sent some texts and emails.

If you were driving, you navigated distances, speed, traffic lights and pedestrians while listening to music or a podcast. However, if you had to find a new way to work because of a train failure or a street being closed off due to an accident, then you would remember. Because you had to get out of the auto-pilot mode, re-focus and make a new plan.

Routines like 'grab-underwear-and-socks' and 'go-to-work' are mainly created along mental pathways in an area of your brain called the basal ganglia. This part of the brain is associated with other highly habitual actions like driving, route selection, and triggering habitual responses when faced with specific stimuli (for example, the way you react when someone throws a punch at you: would you react by closing your eyes and getting hit in the face, or would you keep your eyes open while dodging the aggressor's punch? The way you react can be changed with practice, making it an automatic routine). Re-member the brain is a computer, routines are your cache. You don't have to type in the same set of search words every time to get to a web page. You don't have to remember how to get dressed. For simplicity, from now onwards, I'll refer to those routines that the basal ganglia runs on automatic as 'autopilot'.

When most of your daily routines go on autopilot, your brain saves mental space, energy and time. You are then able to direct your attention to where it is needed most. When you go on autopilot with getting dressed, showering, getting to work or doing something else that is highly familiar, your attention can be directed to something unrelated to what you are doing, like thinking about a work project or just listening to a song or podcast.

⬤ **It's in the space in between routines that you can create moments to relax and truly enjoy yourself.**

While functioning on autopilot is mediated by the basal ganglia, making choices and planning are mediated by the cortex. So, if you have to come up with a new route to work and find yourself in an unfamiliar part of town, your cortex will get to work, and this is high energy and attention consuming. You won't be able to pay attention to a podcast and plan a new route through rush hour traffic at the same time.

The ability to transfer decision making away from the cortex (actually thinking about what you are doing) towards the basal ganglia (operating on autopilot) requires some degree of repetition, and the amount of repetition will vary between individuals and tasks.

One way to reduce decision-making fatigue and preserve willpower for decisions that matter is by making positive behaviours, or essential tasks, routine parts of our day. When something becomes routine, we no longer have to think about it — it's set on autopilot. It's in the browsing history. The favorites tab is already open.

A routine can be as uncomplicated as simplifying our closets. High performers tend to wear the same few combinations of clothes. They quickly grab-and-match from their tidy and organized wardrobe. Like Andreas, 35, hedge fund manager, who has in his closet just twelve shirts, five ties and four pairs of trousers, all in colors that coordinate. He doesn't need to wonder what to wear at 6am, and he saves a lot of time and decision fatigue in the first hours of the day.

The less you have to think about doing something, the more likely it is that you'll actually do it. Instead of having to use willpower to decide whether or not you'll work out that day, you simply work out because that's part of your morning routine. That's the power of routines. They need to be firmly set in place because routines lose all their power if they are vague.

We generally can't control what goes on in the middle of a day, but we can usually control how we begin and end the day, therefore evening and morning routines are key. If we decide to get up whenever, and do whatever, and go to bed whenever, nothing of value is accomplished.

Aim to wake up at the same time every day and try to go to bed at the same time every night. It may sound boring to many people at first, but structure and consistency are crucial to success. We cannot brush and floss our teeth once in a while and hope they stay free of cavities and plaque. Relying on our routines shouldn't be perceived as boring. 'Boring' would be looking up and finding ourselves in the same place five years from now, or even in a worse place: with a few extra pounds of unwanted body fat, reduced muscle flexibility and joint mobility.

• • •

Let's look at Helen, 37, corporate lawyer, who on week-days has well-defined morning and night routines.

Morning routine on Monday/Wednesday/Friday

5.15am: Arise, drink a glass of water, make a smoothie and coffee.

5.30am: Empty bowels, put gym clothes on.

5.45am: Leave for the gym close to her workplace. While on the train, she reviews her schedule and goals for the day.

6.15am: Start workout (often a class).

7.20am: Shower at the gym, get ready to go to work.

8.00am: Have breakfast and a coffee at the canteen at work.

8.30am: Start working.

Morning routine on Tuesday/Thursday

5.15am: Arise, drink a glass of water, make a smoothie and coffee.

5.30am: Empty bowels, have a shower, get ready to go to work.

6.30am: 45 minutes used to either read the news or a book.

7.15am: On her way to work, she reviews her schedule and goals for the day.

8.00am: Have breakfast and a coffee at the canteen.

8.30am: Start working.

Night routine on weekdays

8.00pm: Have dinner with her partner. 1–2 days a week she sees a friend for dinner.

9.30pm: Have a hot shower followed by drinking herbal tea.

10.00pm: Read a book or listen to a podcast.

10.30pm: Lights out.

During the working week, Helen tries to be structured at the start and the end of the day because she has an unpredictable job with long meetings and last-minute crises. Working out during the day is rarely possible. One of Helen's priorities is having time and energy to enjoy her partner's company at night, hence working out after work is not feasible. This is why she includes working out into her morning routine as it is the only part of the day that she has control over.

Basic Routines

#1 — Training in the morning

In order to stick to that morning routine, working out pretty much every weekday, Helen makes sure that when the alarm goes off, her mental and physical resources are directed exclusively (or as much as possible) towards executing actions that are integral to the routine, so she is not distracted by environmental or logistical factors. Her tricks include:

- The night before, she prepares her training kit and lays it out on the chair next to her bed, with her shoes ready to be worn.
- She prepares her bag with her clothes for work and her make-up case.
- In the evening, she takes a warm shower then she drinks herbal tea.
- She sets the alarm on her phone, and she puts her phone far from the bed. This way she will need to get up to grab her phone and stop the alarm.
- Once in bed, she tries to fall asleep as quickly as possible, which is key for getting enough sleep (as we will see in chapter 4).
- As soon as she hears the alarm, she gets up and dresses in her training clothes immediately. She ignores the inner dialogue that will try to bring her back to bed.
- She knows which type of workout she will do. Knowing what to do is liberating, and it helps the task feel easier.
- She leaves the house and catches the 5.45am train.

Helen reduces her mental effort to a minimum to get up and go for a workout while making every single action trigger another action, like a chain reaction. The same way, if you want to floss your teeth more often, you cannot rely on the fact that waking up with the intention to floss your teeth will make it happen. You better keep your floss next to your toothbrush, then you will reach for it and floss your teeth automatically after brushing. It will become an effortless task that you will do without having to expend precious willpower, especially in the morning.

Win the morning, win the day. As 34% of my clients' cancellations are caused by work issues, it's clear that getting to a workout in the morning would decrease the number of missed training sessions drastically. That's why most successful people try to work out in the morning, as this ensures they accomplish their task before the chaos and interruptions of the work day get in the way, when time and willpower are diminished towards the end of the day.

#2 — Eating at the same place

Another way to rely on routine over willpower for repetitive actions is narrowing your lunch choices to only 2, and alternating them day after day. Because the last thing you want is to let your mood and feelings decide what to eat after a hectic morning.

Remember, the most successful clients, regardless of whether their goal is muscle gain or fat loss, eat the same few meals over and over again during their working week. And, whenever possible, it makes sense doing it at the same few places. For example, Helen eats at a nice café close to her workplace.

> She selects 1-2 options from the menu that suit her current diet plan.
> The staff know that she doesn't want bread on the table or sugary sauces like ketchup. She doesn't have to worry about the menu or the temptation of the bread on the table, she can phone her loved ones up or read an article to unwind.
> After she's eaten her healthy meal, she can then go back

to work mentally recharged while feeling on top of her diet.

 ▸ Having the same meals during weekdays helps her keep track of her diet, making it easier to adjust or correct when necessary, whilst consuming less willpower. Remember willpower is a finite commodity each day.

#3 — Meal planning

No matter which diet you follow (Paleo diet, Ketogenic diet, Mediterranean diet or just trying to avoid refined sugar and packaged foods), when you have to put a meal together it is better to rely on a routine which is a developed mental pathway that fits your current diet that, according to its old meaning of 'way of living', should fit into your lifestyle to keep you healthy and productive.

For example, Mark has a job which requires him to travel often between London, New York, LA and others filming locations. Intensive intercontinental travelling causes jet lag, dehydration and lack of sleep — three factors which lead to craving 'comfort food' like sweets and crisps. That's why Mark cannot afford to rely on his feelings and willpower to manage food choices.

When he is either at the buffet of the executive club lounge or at the corporate café at the airport, Mark follows a specific routine. Remember the basal ganglia where the routines that make us go on autopilot are stored? Mark has developed a mental pathway as a habit for his meal choices, wherever the situation. This mental-effort-free routine makes him more likely to stick with his 'wholefood plant-based, slow carb' diet. Mark's routine is:

A. One choice of protein (meat, fish, eggs, soy), one palm-sized portion of his choice.

B. At least three sources of non-starchy vegetables (broccoli, cabbage, cauliflower, peppers, mushrooms, tomatoes etc.), one palm-sized portion of each choice.

C. One choice of starchy vegetables (potatoes, rice, wheat, barley, rye, oats, sweetcorn, beans, lentils, chickpeas, etc.), One fist-sized portion.

D. Condiment: One tablespoon of extra virgin olive oil.

E. At least two glasses of water

Whenever Mark needs to make his own plate, or when grabbing food on-the-go from the fridge of a café, he makes his balanced meal following this mental pathway of A-B-C-D-E. Whatever diet you are following, you need to build a quick and mental-effort-free pathway for every time you need to put a meal together, no matter the situation.

#4 — Airplane travel

People who travel a lot for work need to implement effective strategies to keep healthy despite a tight travelling schedule. No matter how long the haul, domestic or international, air travel has an impact on energy levels and general health.

First, there is dehydration caused by the air conditioning. Upon exposure to air conditioning, we can lose up to 1.5 litres of water for every 3 hours of air travel. So, if you are flying London to New York (approximately 5.5 hours), you could lose about 3 litres of water. Combine that with the fact that we lose an additional glass of water per every glass of wine or coffee we drink, and you can see the final effect taking shape. By the time you land you are likely to be dehydrated, especially your brain, which is mostly made of water.

Having a dehydrated brain causes severe fatigue and headaches, and this is even before the jet lag kicks in. When the brain is dehydrated, we don't feel up for working out and instead we are likely to crave sugary or starchy comfort food.

The following days, jet lag will be a difficult opponent to fight against, because for every day that we are in a different time zone, we readjust about one hour per day. Every time I go to LA for work, it takes me 8 days to readjust to London time, since London is 8 hours ahead of LA. Although you might have noticed that it is easier to adapt to a new time zone when flying westward compared to flying eastwards, no matter if west or east, jet lag affects the brain, organs, and the various apparatus of the body.

Our bodies are programmed to run on cycles known as circadian rhythms, and even little changes in our routine caused by travelling long distances — or even as minimal as changing shift work — disrupts those rhythms and impacts energy levels.

Considering all the above, it is not surprising that very often people plan to work out immediately after landing, or the following day first thing, but then they don't end up doing it. Although they keep bringing their training kit with them to business trip after business trip, they rarely — if ever — use it. To maintain a healthy lifestyle, it's important to use specific strategies and incorporate them into a *travelling routine*. Routine helps reduce the hampering effects of dehydration and jet lag, therefore making working out more likely to happen once we've arrived at our destination, instead of wasting days with no action. A few tips to help you develop a travelling routine are:

- **Before the trip**: book the same hotel. When you are familiar with the same environment and same faces, you spend less mind space adapting to the new environment. This will give you more inspiration to work out. Try to book a hotel with a gym. If that is not possible, you can still pre-book the closest local gym, or go for a run.
- **At the airport**: purchase (or bring from home) a meal and snacks for the flight. For example, a few small bags of various seeds and nuts that are full of fibre, protein, omega-3 and omega-6 fats, which will make you feel satisfied. Drink a large glass of water before boarding.
- **In flight**: Drink one glass of water per hour of flying. If you plan to sleep for 3-4 hours, drink two glasses of water beforehand. You won't go to the toilet as often as you might think. Ask for a bottle of water from the flight attendants. Avoid alcohol and coffee as they both have a diuretic effect.
- **Once you have landed and checked-in at the hotel**: if you have never been in that hotel before, go and have a look at the gym. Getting familiar with that environment will ease the process. Also, knowing which pieces of training equipment are available will help you put together the training routine that you will do just a few minutes later.
- Go to your room, get changed.
- If you don't have a selection of training routines on your phone, take a moment to write one before hitting the gym.

I normally use a notepad next to my bed. Keep it simple and short.

▶ Go train.

The following day you will feel more positive, refreshed and able to handle jet lag much better.

#5 — Weekend routines

For most people, their weekend schedule is different to their work week schedule. For example, taking the children to various sports activities or school parties, having lunch with the in-laws, meeting friends for dinner and staying up until late at social events, make every weekend schedule pretty unique. The variable schedule of each weekend can get in the way of doing physical activity, eating healthily and getting good quality sleep, therefore making it very easy to lose momentum and disrupt your weekly routine from day one. In this scenario, the capacity to *plan in advance* is key. We will talk more extensively about this in chapter 6.

When routines become shackles

Routines streamline your day by reducing decision fatigue, saving your precious mental energy to be used for more demanding tasks. However, there are types of routines that can have the opposite effect, instead disrupting your day. These types of routines lead to varying degrees of unhealthy addictions that complicate and hinder healthy living.

These unhealthy routines are activated by a cue, and at the

end of the routine, there is a reward. The reward reinforces the cue at every single step following this loop:

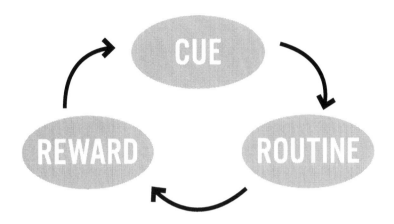

We like to repeatedly engage in activities that we find rewarding — these can be physical or emotional (or both), and are often related to food, sex, social interaction (status, money, etc.) or mood-altering chemicals (alcohol, tobacco, drugs). Often, we associate a particular cue with a desirable outcome — when the outcome is something harmful, we often try to engage willpower to dissociate a cue with participation in an activity that would lead to a specific outcome, but that is very hard. Remember willpower is not an unlimited resource and is often depleted by the time the cues are triggered. A classic example is an irresistible urge experienced by a smoker to smoke when seeing another person light a cigarette.

This is a result of a strong association built up in the brain, between a cue (sight of a cigarette), a routine/behaviour (lighting up a cigarette) and reward (a nicotine rush).

43

Similar examples are:

▶ Compulsive smartphone checking: the cue is the 'ping' or sight of an unchecked message that activates the routine *checking the phone*. The reward is the feeling of belonging/engagement with a person/group/social network post.

▶ Craving sugary foods: the cue is the sight/smell of a cake or pastry that activates the routine *eating the sugary food*. The reward is the blood sugar rush.

Cues and rewards can also be emotional. They don't have to involve a sound, sight or smell trigger. Emotional cues are usually states of anxiety/sadness/boredom, which we aim to displace by engaging with something readily available and immediately distracting from the feeling we don't want to experience.

Unhealthy routines can be very subjective. I personally am more likely to overeat when I'm bored and uninspired, like when I'm working on something dull, such as my accountancy at home. I struggle to keep my head out of the fridge and kitchen cupboards. For other people, anger or sadness leads to overeating. In both scenarios, the reward is the temporary emotional release from the feeling we didn't want to experience.

When a top performer is surrounded by colleagues and acquaintances who use tobacco or alcohol as a way of managing stress or maintaining their performance levels, then it is easy to be drawn into these behaviours for social reasons. Combined with a demanding job, business travel and a busy family life, these behaviours can overwhelm even the best-intentioned individual.

Unhealthy routines are more likely to form during business travel and family holidays, when there is a drastic change of routine. Eating too many refined carbs, smoking a few more cigarettes than normal, or drinking a couple of whiskeys after dinner, can quickly become the new norm. Upon their return to normal life, people often struggle for days, if not weeks, to eliminate these new unhealthy routines and get back into their previous healthy lifestyle.

This is a source of many problems, the most common being loss of motivation and body fat gain. That's when unhealthy routines spiral into time-wasting and energy-draining habits. It is clear that the amount of time necessary to eliminate the new unhealthy routines after *a break* is critical to maintaining a healthy lifestyle. Therefore, whenever your routine is broken by work trips, holidays or long weekends, getting back into a proper routine from day one is key. In order to do that, it's important to identify the new unhealthy routine that is disrupting your day and your quest towards your goals; then take action and try to break it. Identify the cues, and then replace the detrimental cue–reward cycle to stop the unhealthy routine.

45

How to break unhealthy routines

The most common approach that people use to break an unhealthy routine is resisting the actions and behaviors of routine. Although once the routine is triggered then it is often too powerful to break and willpower struggles against it.

That's why trying to stop smoking by simply trying not

to reach for the cigarettes in your pocket is quite impossible. It would be better to resist or eliminate the cue (sight/smell of cigarette) and reward (find a substitution to nicotine) rather than attempting to just resist.

For example, you may want to stop snacking on bread at the restaurant while waiting for your meal. This is such a fattening routine. The cue is seeing the bread in front of you on the table. What can you do? **Eliminate the cue**: Immediately after you arrive at the restaurant, as soon as the waiter has taken you to the table, ask for olives, pickles or nuts. It sounds easy to do but in fact it is really difficult. You will forget a few times. Keep doing it, and every time you manage to do it, take a moment and focus on your sense of accomplishment. That's the **reward** of this new routine: a sense of accomplishment, feeling in control, an upgrade in self-esteem. Practice a few times, and you will start doing it automatically, without thinking about it.

The most effective strategies to avoid or correct an unhealthy routine *do not use willpower* once the routine started — once the cue has been triggered — but instead identify and eliminate (or anticipate) the cue, and override or replace the reward with a healthier alternative.

The key steps are:
1) **Identify cues and rewards.** Observe your behavior and find patterns. Become aware of how you react in hot-blooded situations.
2) **Choose a reaction ahead of time.** Plan ahead, to avoid and eliminate the cues that make you vulnerable.
3) **Reward** yourself with something else.

STRONG STRATEGIES

Have consistent daily, morning and night routines. As part of them:

▶ During the working week, wake up at the same time. At least 30 minutes earlier than the last possible moment.

▶ When you eat out at lunch, go to the same two or three places where you know the menu.

▶ When on-the-go, use the same mental pathway to put together a meal.

▶ Prepare your gym bag/running kit the night before.

▶ At night, set the kitchen ready to make breakfast the following morning.

▶ When you make dinner, cook enough for your lunch to pack up for the following day.

▶ After a holiday or work trip, try to get back into your regular routine from day one, or as soon as possible. And, more than anything else, it is the first workout that will help you reset and get back into your fitness routine, correct eating and good quality sleep.

3
SLEEP

Modern society is plagued with chronic sleep-deprivation — less than seven hours of sleep a night. The combination of many factors contributes to sleep-deprivation: a high degree of integration between work, leisure and life; the backlight of television and computer screens; longer commutes; and a host of other aspects of modern life. Lack of sleep causes more than just impaired focus, bad moods, irritability and anxiety. Lack of sleep weakens the immune system in many ways. One of them is atherosclerosis, which is an increase of plaque in your capillaries, which are the smallest blood vessels. This increase of plaque puts you at risk of heart disease and strokes. Another is Alzheimer's, which is bad news for those who aim to live a long life with a sharp brain.

- **Getting enough quality sleep is essential to keep strong in body and mind and sustain a long, healthy life.**

In chapter 1, I explained that 26% of cancellations for personal training sessions are caused by feeling run-down due to poor sleep. In my experience, together with an overcrowded mind space, lack of sleep is the second most hampering factor on the daily quest of a busy individual to keep healthy.

Along with demanding lifestyles and high stress, most people consider sleep a passive and inactive condition that the body uses to restock its energy supplies. Quality sleep is sacrificed, believing the brain shuts down. In fact, our brain is very active while we sleep.

The reasons you need good quality sleep

Defragmentation. During the day, our brain collects a massive amount of data that get re-processed and re-organised while we sleep. That's when new routines are consolidated, memories are strengthened and new associations between events are made. When we don't sleep well, we struggle to remember certain facts/conversations/meetings, and on which days and what time they occurred.

Waste disposal. The brain is the only organ of the human body that cannot get rid of the waste (as a buildup of chemicals and toxins) it accumulates during the metabolic processes while awake. The brain can only get rid of its toxic waste while it is asleep. Therefore, if we stay awake for too long, or we don't sleep enough, our brain accumulates too many chemicals and toxins that hamper our thinking power, making us slow and sluggish, and increases our chances of making poor decisions and mistakes.

High testosterone, low cortisol. Quality sleep keeps testosterone (a.k.a. the 'muscles and sex hormone') high and the cortisol (a.k.a. the 'stress and fat' hormone) low. Cortisol and testosterone are antagonists. When cortisol levels rise, testosterone levels fall. This causes loss of muscle mass and a low sex drive. Getting enough quality sleep is necessary to developing and keeping muscle mass, and is the greatest natural aphrodisiac. The better sleep we have, the lower the cortisol hormone, which is key to keeping physically strong. Cortisol contributes to fat production and hampers the immune system. Cortisol not only creates subcutaneous fat, retaining a lot of water under our skin making us feel flabby and heavy, it also makes our brain foggy.

Synchronised circadian rhythms. The circadian rhythm is our 24-hour internal clock that runs in the background of our brain and cycles between sleepiness and alertness at regular intervals.

51

Those times can be different if we are naturally a night owl or a morning person. Natural light in particular regulates circadian rhythms and with it a cascade of connected events: our hormone production, body temperature, blood pressure, alertness and bowel movements. These, and even our mood, all fluctuate with the passing of the hours of the day.

Think about the ghastly experience that is jet lag — we discussed this in the travel segment. It is caused by the body being out of sync with the world around it. In the short-term, body clock disruption affects memory formation and focus. In the long-term it increases the risk of diseases, quality of life and even life expectancy.

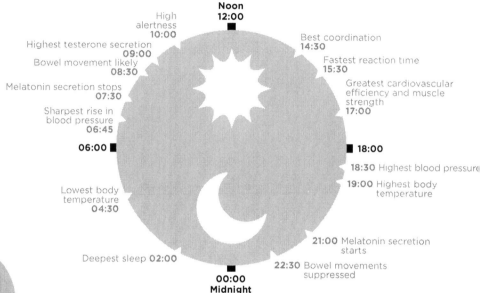

Modern life dynamics clash with our natural circadian rhythm. A few examples of these clashes are:

⟩ When you don't have a consistent morning routine, you get up exhausted and rush to work. Apart from missing time to create mind space to focus and prepare for the busy day ahead, your time for normal body functions and efficient elimination is drastically reduced or postponed to 'sometimes, maybe' during the day. The longer you hold it, the more the toxins are retained, causing bloating and low energy.

⟩ 9am and 12pm: the time of highest testosterone secretion and high alertness, which evolved to force physical effort for hunting and gathering is at 9am and 12pm. That's why doing some cardiovascular activity in the morning on an empty stomach is very effective. Spending calories before eating means you need to 'earn' your meal. Whenever you are too busy or too tired for morning exercise, you are wasting that hormonal trigger, evolved by nature to 'deserve' break-fast. Instead, it's very common to have a sugary breakfast that didn't require any physical effort. The body is confused and the metabolism is messed up.

▶ 3.30pm and 5pm: This is the best time for muscle and strength coordination, designed to help chase a bigger meal. However, during that time you are more likely to be stuck in a chair doing some repetitive work at your desk. That's when the afternoon slump hits you, making you likely to crave sugary and processed comfort food. Again, without having to 'earn' it with physical effort.

▶ 9pm: Melatonin secretion starts. Melatonin is the sleep hormone regulated by light and darkness, so its secretion prepares the body for sleep. Melatonin secretion is hampered by late nights at work, high caffeine consumption during the day, alcohol, electronic devices until late (the 'blue' light that is ubiquitous in the screens around us is mistaken by the body to be daylight). The sleep signals are interrupted.

▶ 11pm: The third alertness window. If you don't go to bed by then (11ish, as it fluctuates with the seasons and latitudes) you get a cortisol push that can keep you awake until 2-3am.

That's a difficult moment to keep strong against cravings for sugary comfort food.

Other factors that disrupt your circadian rhythm are:

▶ Your kids who keep waking you up, noisy neighbours, checking your work emails or social media during the night, the jet lag after a business trip or holiday.

▶ Social jet lag. This phenomenon is so named because it's usually due to people getting out of routine over the weekend, often eating at unusual times, staying awake for longer at night, and a high likelihood of drinking. The side-effects really do mirror jet lag. It's like if you fly on a Friday evening from Paris to New York, or from Los Angeles to Tokyo, and on Monday you fly back. Your circadian biological clock would be de-synchronised with your current time zone. Those individuals who experience social jet lag are more likely to crave sugary foods, consume more caffeine, drink more alcohol, smoke and cancel or skip training.

A life regulated by solid nights' sleep is essential to sustain and maintain a high level of productivity during a demanding day. Together with keeping available mind space, relying on routines, getting enough quality sleep is necessary to streamline your busy day and keep you strong with decisions and feelings.

How do we know that we are not getting enough quality sleep?

How much sleep we need is subjective, although having less than six hours a night demolishes the immune system, increases the chances of catching annoying colds, disrupts blood sugar levels (therefore triggering cravings for sugary foods), and in the long-term contributes to developing more serious brain diseases like Alzheimer.

The amount of sleep you need can be determined by the amount that allows you to be awake, alert and focused during the day. How do you know that you are not getting enough quality sleep? Your body sends you signals to warn you that your mental and physical health is weakening, and that you need to pause to get quality rest. According to a survey I did among my clients, the most common signals that they use as a warning are:

- Lack of balance, clumsiness, tripping while walking
- Find themselves staring at nothing
- Find themselves shaking their head and feeling negative
- Headaches
- Pressure behind swollen eyes
- Sore throat
- Sore glands around the neck
- Cold sores (herpes simplex virus)
- More frequent recurrent colds
- Stiffness on hamstrings, lower back, mid-back, neck and shoulders. A tension that stretching doesn't ease

- Irritability, loss of temper, short answers to co-workers and family members
- Recurrent cravings for foods high in added sugar
- Loss of sex-drive

Before moving to the best strategies for improving the quality of your sleep, I'd like to focus on a key factor, which is the speed at which you fall asleep. This speed is determined by the capacity to control our thoughts, because *a restless mind struggles to fall asleep.*

A restless mind struggles to fall asleep; the more you let your thoughts run wild, the more you will toss and turn. A tired body with a clear mind falls asleep easier than a body that has been resting in a chair for 12 hours but with a tired and overcrowded mind. That's why when you are on holiday, after a big day of skiing or hiking, it is far easier to fall asleep compared to the middle of the work week, when your mind struggles to switch off. The key is being able to shut down the inner dialogue as soon as you reach the pillow, otherwise you risk staying awake for hours, checking the time and your phone.

It is difficult to control inner dialogue at night, especially if you have let it go unchained during the day. Through my daily interaction with world-class performers, I have come to appreciate how they have an 'action mentality'. They are strategists and problem solvers, hence they are constantly planning ahead to maximise resources and obtain the highest results. Their minds are constantly forecasting possible problems and solutions before they even happen.

For example, do you ever think about the dinner you will

have later on with your partner while you're still at work? And then a few hours later, while you are with your partner you are thinking about your next workout at the gym (or your next golf/tennis/football match with your friends). And the following day while working out (or playing sport) you are thinking about the next big work project.

This constant projecting of thoughts to short-term future events becomes a routine that is hard to notice and difficult to break. The risk is that one forgets to pay attention to what is actually happening right here and right now. This means missing the opportunity to enjoy precious moments with the people who really matter. But even more than that, it could mean being in a state of constant tension.

Our mind can be either our strongest asset or the most hampering factor in our attempt to keep a healthy lifestyle. When too much is going on and we are tired, then the anticipation of a task in the immediate future can trigger anxiety and negative inner dialogue. For example, sometimes I have received texts from clients 30-60 minutes before our session saying: *'I'm not sure I can handle an hour session today, can we finish 15 minutes earlier?'* to which I agree. But then, as it always — honestly, always — happens, after a 45 minute session the client says 'I'm actually ok now, can we carry on?'

The fear of discomfort pre-exercise is always higher than during the exercise. And mental struggle is always more difficult to manage than physical struggle. After the session they always feel better, with a clearer mind, steady mood, great sense of achievement and they normally say after stretching 'I'm glad I didn't cancel today. I feel better now.'

Every person is different, and while I don't normally suffer from discomfort or anxiety about an event that is just about to happen, I surely do for an event that will happen in the near future. For example, when I check my diary for the following day and I see 8—10 sessions booked, plus a few telephone calls, plus my workout, then I can feel a sense of anxiety for a day that looks too long, too hectic. But I know the trick that works for me, which is focusing solely on the first task of the day as I know that slowly everything will take care of itself, client after client, telephone call after call, email after email, my workout, my meals, etc.

In any case, it seems that staying in the moment and focusing on the next important task to tackle is better than letting the mind go unchained creating (most of the time) unjustified negative inner dialogue and anxiety.

I've noticed that my clients who are able to come to the gym and focus solely on the training session, leaving work and family issues 'outside', are the ones most satisfied with the quality of their sleep. Perhaps it is not a coincidence, and it might come down to their capacity not only to **stay in the moment,** and focus on the here and now, but also to **compartmentalise,** which is the capacity to separate thoughts into sections and not allow those sections to mix together. People who are somehow able to compartmentalise their thoughts are able to fall asleep anywhere and at any time. For example, during their intercontinental business trips, or using short half an hour naps during the day. Being able to 'compartmentalise' and focus solely on the next most important task with mindfulness is key for a good night's sleep.

Another common trait of successful sleepers is that when something happens to them, for example either falling on the street or receiving bad news, they **move from the denial stage to the acceptance stage** very quickly. This way, they are able to readjust their schedule with ease. Somehow, they see the big picture and **put things in perspective**. Most of the stress comes from the way we respond to situations, not the way life is. When we adjust our perspective, we see the situation from a different angle and we can give a different, more rational response to it. For example, Suzanne, 39, project manager in investment banking — when she feels overwhelmed due to a crisis at work, she tries to keep calm and think 'Am I having a breakdown or a breakthrough?' That is the moment when she manages to keep calm, take one step back to see the big picture and make the right next important decision. In general, those people who are able to pause and put things in perspective are more likely to control their inner dialogue, to keep anxiety at bay and also to fall asleep quickly.

Conscious breathing

At the end of a long busy day during which you have been going full-speed, at night you forget to slow down and you go to bed with your mind on the mental expressway. What can happen is that your thoughts will turn to the next problem to solve tomorrow at work. Needless to say, this results in a lack of sleep and turns into an edgy, anxiety-filled and restless ordeal. When this happens, how do you think you will start your next action-packed day? Anxious. Which will likely affect your day

59

in a way that you will go to bed at full-speed again.

There are many systems that teach us how to focus on the here and now, while controlling thoughts and feelings. These are the ones that I have found to be most effective for the top performers I consult: meditation, yoga, pad work and sparring for ring-sports and martial arts, then an ice bath and Cryotherapy. These disciplines and tasks have a common factor: *conscious breathing*. You literally cannot do any of them without focusing on your breathing.

In Ashtanga and Vinyasa yoga, each movement has a breath, and each breath has a count. This forces you to stay in the moment and focus on what you are doing, without thinking about anything else. In ring-sports and martial arts, every single strike, block, catch, hold, step and the other movements are timed with your breath to optimise speed and stamina. While you are doing an ice bath and Cryotherapy, you really need to focus on your breath to stay calm, slow down the heart rate, waste as little heat as possible and get through the session.

Focusing on your breathing breaks the inner dialogue made up of those persistent cyclical thoughts that trigger anxiety. Breathing brings mindfulness. Do you breathe while working out? Do you breathe while having sex? You would be surprised how most people don't. I tell you because I noticed very often while teaching exercise techniques, either with free weights or kickboxing, that people tend to hold their breath. And if you hold your breath while learning, you'll need more time to learn and master the technique because your inner dialogue is getting in the way.

People who focus on their breath learn much faster, as

they are present in the moment, in a state of both relaxation and readiness. Breathing lowers the heart rate and blood pressure, and stimulates the parasympathetic nervous system which triggers the body to relax. In addition to being a stress-reliever, deep breathing promotes concentration and strengthens the immune system. After you do any activity that forces you to pay attention to your breathing, you will feel mentally rested and calm. Anxiety is reduced, perhaps even completely gone. You might have different disciplines/sports/tasks that work for you in the same way, like swimming or ballet dancing — that is perfectly fine as long as you reach that level of tranquility afterwards. That's the state to aim for in order to fall asleep quickly. How can you use breathing techniques to reproduce that effect of calmness and tranquility whenever you need to? You can practice equal breathing:

Equal breathing

Inhale through the nose for a count of four, then exhale through the nose for a count of four. Once you have got the basics, then you can aim for six to eight counts per breath. The goal is to calm the nervous system, reduce anxiety and slow racing thoughts. Personally, when I feel I'm getting anxious and overwhelmed, I automatically breath deep and slow — it has become an automatic habit. I immediately perceive a sense of calm and control together with a rapid decrease of my heart rate. It's especially effective before bed, but you can do it during the day, while sitting at your desk, at the airport or on the train, or while standing. Pay attention, dizziness is not the goal of this technique. If you feel uncomfortable, tone it down to just a few seconds.

● ● ●

Low quality sleep is not a nighttime disorder, it's a 24-hour disorder. It is clear that sleep is an active task that needs to be looked after as much as physical training and eating correctly. The way you start your day and navigate through it will determine how you end it. If you start your day calm, and manage to get through it calm, you will likely end it calm and tranquil. If you start your day messy and agitated you will likely end it messy and agitated. Having consistent morning and night routines, together with the capacity to practice conscious breathing, stay in the moment, compartmentalise and put things in perspective, is key to getting quality sleep for a long and healthy life.

62

STRONG STRATEGIES

Have a consistent morning routine:

▶ *Create blank time for yourself.* Wake up between 30-60 minutes before you could to avoid doing everything in a rush since the early minutes of the day. That time will allow you either to have breakfast, do a workout, or process your emotions and thoughts through meditation or morning writing. This will also help to manage occasional last-minute transport issues, making you feel in control of your day and less anxious. When you start work with that sense of control and focus, you won't need to rely on as much caffeine and you will be less likely to crave that sweet treat pick-me-up at 10am.

▶ *Work out in the morning*. This reduces the effects of last-minute issues during the day that get in the way of your fitness schedule. It cuts out any anxious thoughts about finding time to work out, especially if you are having a busy day. It eliminates the late evening post-workout adrenaline rush that hinders falling asleep quickly.

63

▶ *Have a breakfast free of added sugar*. If you start your day with a meal high in refined sugars and/or refined flours (most common are wheat, corn, rice and potatoes) you will have a sugar-spike in your bloodstream. This will trigger a cascade of events that will get you stuck into a sugary food craving cycle that results in the over-production of the insulin hormone. Insulin is not only a fattening factor, but also an energy weakening, mood-swinging factor and sleep disruptor.

Mindfulness and compartmentalization. No matter how big the day ahead seems, stay calm, use conscious breathing to keep anxiety at bay and focus on the next important action.

Avoid drinking caffeine after 2pm or at least 8 hours prior to bedtime (earlier if you're sensitive to it). Consider that many energy drinks contain caffeine. This, combined with other ingredients (e.g. Guarana or Taurine) enhances the effect of caffeine even more, and caffeine is also a diuretic that will make you wake up often at night, hampering the quality of your sleep. Today you can track the quality of your sleep with many smartphone applications, so you can see how many times you have awakened.

Get 15 minutes of sun a day whenever possible. No matter if it's summer or winter, 15 minutes of sunlight exposure on your arms or legs is enough to produce enough vitamin D for the day. Vitamin D, among other beneficial effects, improves the quality of your sleep.

During the day stay active and on the move. Spending many hours on a chair staring at the monitor is connected with cravings rich in sugars, increasing the chances that you'll give in and start an energy-draining sugar craving cycle that will make you feel feverish, tired and negative, therefore disrupting your capacity to fall asleep quickly.

Use power naps. Daytime naps help the brain process information that's hidden from conscious awareness. Short periods of sleep are thought to enhance aspects of memory and thinking. Most of the time, after a power nap you are able to see previously challenging problems as much easier to overcome.

Have dinner at least two hours before bedtime.
Your guts also have a bedtime and eating food too late can keep your digestive system awake. No matter which diet plan you are following, if you suffer from insomnia you might need to investigate whether red meat and cheese (which often trigger invigorating effects) are exciting you rather than pacifying your system. The best supplements for better sleep are magnesium and vitamin D.

Avoid alcohol. Having alcohol at night might give that misleading sense of deserved relaxation after a hectic day. In fact, you are more likely to wake up during the night feeling anxious, then struggle to fall back to asleep.

After dinner, have a consistent bedtime routine.
In chapter 2 we have seen how routines are a very powerful instrument for reducing decision fatigue and getting important things done automatically. Effective bedtime routines may include:

- Eliminate, or at least dim, computer screens and TVs, at least one hour before bed.
- Have a caffeine-free drink. Herbal tea with a spoon of raw quality honey just before bed is magical.
- Lay down on a mat and relax, unwind, do some light stretching. Getting to 'touch the floor' has a calming effect.
- Have a warm shower or a bath with magnesium salt.
- Reading.

Go to bed by 10pm. Your body creates a cortisol surge after 11pm to keep you awake, and after that time you will be more likely to crave sugary foods that will cause you to struggle to fall asleep.

Leave the problems and serious talks outside the sleeping environment. Avoid chit-chats/arguments/problem-solving once in the bedroom. The bedroom should be a place only for cuddles, sex (the best sleeping 'pill') and sleeping.

Optimise your sleeping environment. We have seen how, in order to streamline your day, you need to organise your environment in a way that works *for* you and not against you. In order to get to sleep you need an environment that is conducive to sleep. The sleeping environment must be:

▸ *De-cluttered*. The outer environment affects the way you think and feel. It has an effect on your sleep as well.

▸ *Quiet*. If the bedroom is noisy due to outside traffic or the neighbour's TV, use earplugs or listen to a white noise app on your phone and set your alarm. The alarm will interrupt the track so that you wake up whenever you plan to.

▸ *Pitch-dark*. Make it as dark as you possibly can. Block all possible light sources, whether it's a curtain or just pinning up fabric as needed. Especially if you live in a city, light pollution is a big problem. LEDs keep you awake, and these are especially prevalent in hotel rooms: cover them with black secure electrical tape. If it isn't possible to get rid of every source of light, use an eye-mask. When your bedroom is de-cluttered, quiet and pitch dark, it is easier to fall asleep fast.

▶ *Ventilated/clean air*. Heat and high concentrations of CO_2 hamper quality sleep. Even in the winter, keep the window slightly open. If you live in a polluted city, you might consider purchasing an air purifier.

▶ *Quality mattress and pillow*. It is always worth investing some money into a good quality mattress and pillow to give support to the back and neck, for better quality sleep and less chance of waking up with muscles stiffness.

▶ *Use a heavy blanket*. Sleeping under a heavy blanket adds weight, which signals the brain to release chemicals like serotonin, melatonin and dopamine which encourage sleep.

4
SECOND BRAIN

Throughout this book we have covered various strategies that busy individuals use to free up mind space, foster consistent routines and improve their sleep. A key factor that has a direct bearing on the quality of workouts, the capacity to stay sharp, focused and productive during a demanding day is the health of your guts. When a client comes to a session with me and mentions feeling bloated or experiencing bowel issues, I know the session won't be great, because a person with poor gastrointestinal function is never performing at their best. As the cliché goes, we are what we eat — and, by extension, how we digest what we eat. An unhappy gut results in physical and mental fatigue, lack of productivity and general malaise.

● **The health of your guts is a key factor for keeping you highly productive during a demanding day.**

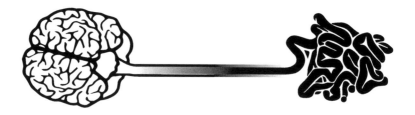

A second brain

Your digestive tract contains around 100 million neurons, in a nervous system that is more complex than the spinal cord. The gut is also home to more neurotransmitters than the brain in your head. Over 90% of your serotonin is found in your enteric nervous system (ENS) — the scientific name for the gut — and several studies show an effect of ENS health on brain and cognitive processes. Several well known co-morbidities have been shown to exist between ENS disorders and psychiatric issues — the most well-known being anxiety and irritable bowel syndrome. Research is also being carried out into why people with autism, attention deficit disorder, dyslexia, obsessive-compulsive disorder, anxiety and depression experience higher incidence of gastric issues than otherwise healthy individuals.

Perhaps it is not a cliché that we should listen to our guts — for it is in there that we 'feel butterflies' when excited or aroused, and we say something is 'gut-wrenching' when we are terrified or grief-stricken, or we 'go with our gut' to make important decisions when in doubt. But of course these are strong feelings, and we don't tend to experience them for long periods of time. Most of the time, a well-functioning organism doesn't feel anything in the gut — the gut simply does it's job of keeping you alive. It is when your guts are troubled, upset or sad that you likely don't feel well. And a damaged gut generally cannot be sorted with a quick fix, like a wristband to support a painful wrist. A damaged gut takes a long time to heal while keeping you tired.

As well as being the home of neurotransmitters, the gut is a veritable jungle of microbes lining the internal surfaces of the whole gastrointestinal tract (and its internal surface area is huge — the size of a tennis court, over 100 times greater than the surface area of your skin). These microbes are the first line of defence, protecting you from harmful agents that enter your system in food and drink.

Good microbes & bad microbes

Some of the inhabitants of your gut cause havoc when they get out of hand. Notably, chlamydia and candida. When out of balance, they cause inflammation of the gut, impeding nutrient absorption. This generally sabotages the effective functioning of a whole number of systems, making the body more susceptible to illness and discomfort. The phenomenon of a 'leaky gut' is a failure of the gastrointestinal tract to contain all harmful agents within it, and successfully push them towards elimination. When gut lining is out of order, substances that usually stay within the gut 'leak' through the gut barrier and are identified as a 'foe' by the immune system. It is currently theorised that this is one way that food allergies develop, and might be the cause of a rising number of reported food allergies and intolerances in adults in the last few decades.

Mild irritation of the gut, and its failure to effectively eliminate useless material, causes irritability, lack of mental acuity and weakens the immune system, exposing the body to illness. You won't function as well as you could be if your gut health was tip-top. The health of your guts determines not only the quality of your general health, but also the way you feel and make decisions during a highly demanding day.

A healthy gut digests food, absorbs nutrients and eliminates waste. This is the stuff of life, it sustains us but it is also influenced by life — the stresses, joys, habits and patterns. Invariably, problems along the digestion/absorption/elimination route are a symptom of underlying issues, and causes unpleasantries that can substantially impede your life. Acid reflux, heartburn, dull skin or skin prone to breakouts, fragile hair and nails, constant hunger, constipation or diarrhea are all very unpleasant to live with. They will all negatively impact your decision-making capability, confidence, temper and — on a daily level — your capacity to exercise and eat well.

What disrupts digestion, absorption and elimination?

1) Foods that upset good microbes and enable bad microbes to thrive.

> **Refined sugars.** These are mostly added to packaged

foods to increase their shelf life and enhance flavour. At least 72 types of refined sugars can be added to food and drink. Examples are: brown sugar, cane sugar, caramel, corn syrup, corn syrup solids, demerara sugar, dextrose, cane juice, fructose, fruit juice concentrate, galactose, glucose, golden syrup, grape sugar, high-fructose corn syrup, lactose, malt syrup, maltose, maple syrup, molasses, muscovado sugar and sucrose.

⟩ **Alcohol.**

⟩ **Artificial sweeteners, artificial colourants, preservatives**. These are heavily used in light drinks and in processed and packaged food, such as aspartame and monosodium glutamate.

⟩ **Pesticides.** Found in fruit and vegetables that are not organic.

⟩ **Antibiotics and hormones**. Could be found in low quality meat and junk food.

2) Food allergies, intolerances and sensitivities

Food allergies are rapid and severe immunological responses to specific foods that cause symptoms such as rashes, wheezing, dizziness, nausea, hayfever, sneezing, and even seizures after exposure to the allergenic foods. If you have any food allergies you would already know by now, as their effects are pretty violent and noticeable.

Food intolerances and sensitivities trigger a range of milder inflammatory reactions, so they are harder to recognise. If every day you ate a food that you were intolerant or sensitive to, you would suffer a series of mild reactions, which would not be severe enough to think something is wrong. Some of the symptoms can appear anything from an hour to a day after consumption of the culprit food.

The symptoms of food intolerances and sensitivities include: reduced focus, mood fluctuations, muscular and joint pain, itchy skin, gastric acid release, bloating, constipation, diarrhea, nasal congestion, low energy and tiredness — which are all easy to get accustomed to. They could even become something you believe is normal. And when a problem becomes normal, we are less likely to recognise it and take action to fix it. Somehow most people struggle to link these mild symptoms to the meal they just had. For example, gastric reflux after eating a cake made with yeast, or mild diarrhea after a latte, three days of constipation following a weekend binging on white bread and pasta, shaky hands after a coffee, sweating after red meat, headache after cheese, fatigue after rice, fruit followed by feelings of being bloated and flatulence.

It is advisable to exclude every possible intolerance or sensitivity that might be affecting the digestive system. Today there isn't a comprehensive test recognised by doctors which could be used to diagnose food intolerances and sensitivities. However, my clients have used a combination of the following to achieve a reasonably high degree of accuracy:

▶ **Keeping a food and energy diary** to discover patterns in changes of energy levels and elimination after you eat a specific food. Once you have noticed a link between low energy/change in mood and a specific food, the next step would be to try an 'elimination diet'. This involves cutting the suspected food out of your diet for at least two weeks and then reintroducing it while monitoring symptoms. It is better to do it under the supervision of your doctor.

▶ **Bioenergetic screening**. This test is not invasive and quick to do, as it consists of holding two electrodes for five minutes. The report works well in combination with the food and energy diary to discover otherwise hidden patterns.

We shouldn't be obsessing over everything we eat. By all means, enjoy an occasional snack that comes out of a packet, or anything you feel is a treat. Do it, and don't feel guilty — but the key here is 'occasional'. The major point is to try and tilt your diet towards foods that do not result in you experiencing bodily sensations that are unpleasant.

Emotional food cravings

Considering the deep link between brain and digestive system it is very important to acknowledge the role of emotion in what we eat. Particularly, to acknowledge that sometimes cravings are a way for us to avoid experiencing emotions that we find unpleasant. Stress, anxiety, shame or guilt can, and frequently do, result in cravings for sugar, salt and alcohol. These cravings will have nothing to do with low blood sugar or gut health, but they will impact blood sugar and gut health. That is to say, you might be driven to eat something because you wish to 'treat' yourself and immerse yourself in the immediate pleasure of food (and avoid the displeasure of an invasive feeling). But the result will be a feeling of guilt afterwards, and quite possibly the incremental weakening of your gut health.

If 'out of the blue' cravings for foods you wish to generally avoid is something you wish to learn more about, I recommend the WWH technique.

The WWH technique

A powerful tool to identify the emotional trigger for your mysterious urge to eat is the WWH (what, where, how) technique. The WWH technique requires you to write down:

- What happened just before the craving?
- Where were you when the sugar craving started?
- How did you feel just before?

Let's see an example:

Jenny, 28, is a PR Manager in the music industry. She used to suffer from cravings for milk chocolate. She said the cravings were happening at different times of the day, without a reason. She used the WWH card for a week and the breakdown was as follows:

On **Tuesday**, Jenny had a craving at 10pm and she ate three milk chocolate bars.
- **What happened just before?** Her 5-year-old kid didn't want to go to bed.
- **Where was she when the craving started?** She was

in the kitchen, where she went straight after her son finally agreed to go to bed.

▶ **How did she feel?** She felt upset with her ex-husband, as he had allowed their son to stay up late at the weekend, hence he'd got into a bad habit.

On **Thursday**, Jenny had a craving at 1pm. She ate two milk chocolate bars from the vending machine just before a meeting.

▶ **What happened just before?** She was told she had to stay in the office for a last-minute meeting with a new client. She had planned to go to the gym at that time. She wouldn't have any available time to work out for the rest of the day due to her family schedule.

▶ **Where was she when the cravings started?** Sitting in the office waiting for the client.

▶ **How did she feel?** She was upset. She also felt she was not in control with her job and life.

From looking at these results, it was clear that the trigger of Jenny's cravings was emotional: anger, frustration and/or sadness. Once Jenny discovered the feelings that trigger her emotional eating, she had to work over how she was reacting to those feelings, using the key steps we have seen in C2 – How to break unhealthy routines (page 45):

1) **Identify cues and rewards.** Observe your behavior and find patterns. Become aware of how you react in hot-blooded situations.

2) Choose a reaction ahead of time. Plan ahead, to avoid and eliminate the cues that make you vulnerable.

3) Reward yourself with something else.

When the cue is emotional (anxiety/sadness/boredom) the reward is *engaging with something readily available and immediately distracting from the feeling that we don't want to experience.* With Jenny, we studied the follow sequence of decisions to take every time she had an emotional food craving.

1. Change scenario/environment (leave the kitchen, or the desk if at work, even briefly) and start a new enjoyable task like going for a short walk in a nice place, talking to a colleague, calling a friend up.

2. If the food craving was still there, drink a glass of water and then eat the least damaging food option available (for her was 72% dark chocolate, or full fat yogurt with strawberries).

Emotional food cravings are hard to manage and they can often disrupt even the best diet plan. There is not magic pill to emotional eating, only a rational approach to it. That's because food brings comfort, like a feeling of safety and control. Once we understand which emotions trigger our cravings, we become aware of our reactions and can tackle the emotional cues head on. The WWH technique helps to do this by making you aware of patterns and behaviours, triggers and reactions. The

WWH technique helps discover the triggers that are unique to every individual. It is important that you find the unique triggers for your food cravings, because *food should never be the remedy to feelings generated by work, family or life problems.*

Obviously certain behaviours could be triggered by issues caused by significant events in life, even events which happened many decades before, and so they would need to be treated by a psychiatrist or psychologist.

My focus as a coach is **not about what happened before**, but instead how I can help you **from now on to move towards** your goals. And from this perspective I invite my clients who struggle with emotional food cravings to keep two mantras in mind:

- ▶ **We are filters**. All of us interpret situations according to previous experiences and current feelings. Most of the time it is *1% what happens and 99% how we react* that makes a difference. In other words, our capacity to take a step back in stressful situations and see the big picture, and to put things in perspective, is key to avoiding (or resisting) emotional food cravings.
- ▶ **Watch the little kid**. Whenever we have an emotional craving, if we could observe our actions from the outside, we would see ourselves looking like a little kid having a tantrum for sweets, crisps or packaged food.

Personally, I know that I have two triggers for emotional eating. My first emotional trigger is boredom. When I have to work on something which I find tedious and uninspiring,

I struggle to keep out of the fridge and the cupboards. I crave savoury snacks, like crisps. To manage this, I try to plan ahead for when I have to work on jobs which I find boring. I fill my fridge with healthy food and avoid working in a café, where I know temptations will be aplenty.

My second emotional trigger is the smell of fresh tomato sauce that makes me feel safe and at home. This is because it reminds me of my childhood, when my mother made fresh tomato sauce from scratch every single morning, and our home was filled with that divine scent. No matter how full I am after a meal, if I smell fresh tomato sauce coming from a restaurant, I feel deceptively hungry for anything with that sauce. This has an easy solution, which is to avoid walking around food courts where I would smell that scent.

Overall, cravings for comfort food are like waves that come and go during the day. Whenever I've just had a meal but after a bit I still crave some food that I know *I'm not supposed to eat*, I know something else is going on. Firstly, I drink a glass of water as the craving could be caused just by dehydration. In fact, most of the time, after having water the craving for that food disappears. If the food craving is still there, I pause and try to understand if it's triggered by me feeling overwhelmed due to overcrowded mind space caused by a hectic day. In that case, I use conscious breathing and I try to relax and de-stress. If the food craving is caused by boredom or tiredness, then I start doing something more interesting and fun to keep my mind busy. When it doesn't work, then I drink a glass of water and eat the best available food option.

STRONG STRATEGIES

▶ Stick to a wholefood, organic-based diet to reduce consumption of refined sugars, artificial sweeteners, artificial colorants, preservatives, pesticides, antibiotics and hormones as much as possible.

▶ Reduce alcohol intake as much as possible and drink lots of water during the day.

▶ Nurture your gut's microbiome by eating non-starchy and high in fibre vegetables (broccoli, cabbage, kale, etc.), and pickles and fermented foods (olives, onions, sauerkraut, kimchi, kefir, kombucha, miso, tempeh, full-fat yogurt).

▶ Find out which foods you might be intolerant and sensitive to, if any, and avoid them.

▶ Get a grip on your emotional eating and use the WWH technique to discover the root of your emotional cravings.

▶ When a food craving comes, pause, breath and think before you eat.

5

SOCIAL EVENTS

Social events centred on food and drink like work dinners, parties and family reunions can disrupt even the best efforts of keeping consistency with a fitness schedule and diet. This is due to the unhealthy food served and the social pressure around drinking alcohol. While the food can be managed with some proactive strategies, it is much harder to avoid drinks placed in our hands by co-workers and friends who expect us to drink with them. Especially in countries like Great Britain, where drinking is deeply ingrained in society as a way to socialise — this social pressure is very difficult to manage.

Drinking can bring two types of pressure:

▶ Direct social pressure, when someone offers you a drink or an opportunity to drink.
▶ Indirect social pressure, when you feel tempted to drink just by being around others who are indulging, even if no one offers you a drink.

I've observed both direct and indirect social pressure affect even individuals with a strong drive and willpower. When there are too many social events of this kind in a row, their capacity to keep strong and rely on their willpower to say, 'No, thank you' diminishes, especially in the last hours of a busy day that drain mental and physical energy. The risk here is giving in and starting a cycle of over-eating and over-drinking that will last for a few days, if not weeks, afterwards.

A frequent reason for missing a workout is being hungover, and most of the time the excess of drinking happens at work or events with family and friends. It is clear that in order to keep up momentum with a fitness schedule and diet, you need to be prepared for these social events. Actions reflect priorities, therefore you need to prepare for every social event exactly like you would do for a presentation at work. You might not want your social life to feel like work, but unfortunately eating and drinking cannot be left to 'let's see how I feel tonight', especially if the following day is busy and you probably won't have much time to work out.

● **Have a strategy for every social event that is centred on food and drinks.**

The following strategies are the ones that I find to be most effective when my clients wish to keep on track with their diet, without compromising their busy lifestyle. The more you apply these strategies, the easier, more effortless and more effective they will feel.

Strong strategies for social events centred on eating

▶ If the event is a sit-down lunch or dinner at a restaurant, research the restaurant's menu online beforehand. If you know what to order, it will be easier to follow your plan without hesitating or ordering impulsively.

▶ If the event is a buffet and you know how hard it is to resist the plate of mini sausages when it's offered directly to you — especially in front of other people who just took some and are looking at you, waiting to share the experience — the best thing is to serve yourself.

▶ If you know the food you will be served is not what you want to eat, don't go there hungry. Have a healthy meal or snack before you arrive to help dull the temptation before it even starts. More importantly, drink a large glass of water before reaching for anything tempting. Staying well hydrated can help minimise feelings of hunger that may trigger you to reach out for tempting foods.

▶ Watch out for random food pushers: food pushers are those people who will try to get you to 'taste' the food they are eating, or they have cooked. It's usually followed by them staring at you as you go from one bite to the other all bug-eyed, waiting for a response. Awkward, I know. The best response is to say politely but firmly: *'Wow, it looks delicious. I would love to, but I am quite full right now, I'll have it later. Thank you.'*

Somehow, giving up certain foods to increase productivity at work or to prepare for a competition are reasons more socially accepted than improving health. Perhaps because the notion of health is quite abstract, it's hard to visualise and perceive until it's lost. Think about it; we normally understand how healthy we were only when we get ill. Probably because we truly recognise the value of health only when it deteriorates.

When you tell people that you want to improve your health, they look at you blank. Instead, try something like; *'Since I have cut out sugar and refined flours I feel my mind is clearer and my energy levels are higher'* or *'I'm preparing for a triathlon/white collar boxing/swimming competition.'* Goal- or results-oriented replies work better than *'I don't want that because it's not healthy'.* People will visualise something tangible that you are putting so much effort in to achieve, and will be more supportive.

You're at a family dinner, and you have already filled your plate with slices of turkey and roasted veggies. Aunty Sue sees you haven't served yourself any stuffing, so she graciously does it for you. You thank her for remembering you love stuffing. Then you push it around on your plate or discreetly dispose of it to make it look like you had some. Sometimes a white lie is preferable to hurting Aunty Sue's feelings. If Aunty Sue insists you try 'just one bite' of her famous fruitcake, you can reply *'I wish I could. But it's probably so delicious that I won't be able to stop at one, so I'd better not even start!'* I know it's not easy. I have an Italian mother, and perhaps you don't have any idea how hard it is saying no to an Italian mother who has just cooked for you. She is pushy, her food is delicious and trust me: you don't want to upset her as life can become difficult for a few days. And still, I had to learn how to say 'no, thanks' with a calm and firm tone, while smiling and keeping eye contact in a way that doesn't show any doubts.

Strong strategies for social events centred on drinking

▶ Between 30mins and 1 hour before the event, eat something with healthy fats like omega-3, omega-6, omega-9: oily fish, meat, eggs, cheese, nuts, seeds, avocado, coconut oil and extra virgin olive oil. These fats slow digestion down and hence delay alcohol absorption. Drink plenty of water — the more hydrated you are, the slower you will get drunk.

▶ The Night Saver. I've learnt this from Ben, 39, an agent for actors and scriptwriters in LA. He relies on the Night Saver as he goes out pretty much every single night to attend various work events. Once Ben arrives at the event, he goes straight to the bar in the most natural way and asks for a glass of water with ice, a straw and lemon or lime. That's the Night Saver, and it pretends to be a vodka and soda, or a gin and tonic in disguise. When Ben finishes it, he gets another Night Saver as before. Remember, serve yourself.

▶ If you decide to have just a few alcoholic drinks, then have a Night Saver for every two alcoholic drinks. For your alcoholic drinks choose one measure of pure forms plus a sugar-free tonic. The purest form of alcohol to drink is a highly purified alcohol with no added sugar, sulphites or additives. Therefore, spirits like vodka, tequila, gin and whisky are much better than champagne, wine, beer and cider. Examples of better drinks to order:

- Triple purified vodka, with fresh orange juice (not from concentrate, to reduce sugar intake as much as possible).
- Gin with soda water and lime.
- Mojito, without sugar. Somehow bartenders find it difficult to change a recipe and often resist. Insist and get what you ask for.

▶ Stick with the same alcoholic drink. The more you mix, the more you get drunk and lose control, and the more painful it will be the following morning. If you start with vodka, carry on with vodka. Tequila especially should not be mixed with other spirits.

▶ If someone gives you an alcoholic drink and you feel stuck, don't panic. Sip once, smile and engage in deep conversation for a bit. Try to leave to put your glass away. If for some reason it is difficult to get out of that conversation, be aware that as soon as you feel the first buzz, it means that your body's detoxification pathways are becoming overwhelmed which means you are getting too drunk. Excuse yourself with a smile and head to the toilets. Pour your alcoholic drink in the toilet, fill your glass with tap water or go to the bar and get a Night Saver.

Overall mind these two key factors:

1) HYDRATION: Your body needs water to eliminate the toxins of drinks via urination. This necessary water comes from your tissue or the water you drink, so better to drink water and avoid getting dehydrated. When the brain is dehydrated you lose your thinking power and sticking with the plan becomes even more difficult. In order to keep hydrated:

> ❭ Drink plenty of water during the day leading up to the event.
> ❭ Drink Night Savers during the event.
> ❭ Drink more water when you get home and before bed. It will ease the effect of the alcohol the following morning.

2) PACING: Whenever you decide to enjoy your alcoholic drinks without using Night Savers, but you still want to avoid being flat out in bed the following day, then pacing (drinking slowly) is key. For example I've learnt from my client Alex, founder of a technology company in the Silicon Valley, to drink beer from a bottle instead of a glass. Not only do you normally drink slower from a bottle, but also in this way colleagues and friends are less able to see how much beer you have left in your bottle, hence they won't keep bringing more drinks to you every time they finish theirs. Learning and keeping to your own drinking pace and not someone else's will keep you in control.

When the night changes direction: success or disaster?

▶ Finally, avoid 'shots time' — the killer of every perfect plan and the best of intentions. How many times have you been doing quite well, having decided to drink slowly, not at all, or stick to just one type of drink? It might go well for a while, until someone, often a very close friend or colleague, decides it's *'shots time'*!

And the way you manage that moment will make a difference between success and disaster...

▶ Outcome 1: Getting up the following day fresh enough to be productive, deliver everything as planned, including working out and eating as planned. SUCCESS.

OR

▶ Outcome 2: Waking up but unable to get up. Having a painful and unproductive day. Unable to work out and craving very unhealthy food. This state of low-energy might continue for a few days. DISASTER.

Although everybody would theoretically choose Outcome 1, in reality, it is tough to avoid Outcome 2. That's because once the shots are lined up in front of our eyes, and everybody picks a glass up while looking at us and smiling, it becomes difficult to say no. Saying *'no, thanks'* to people you're emotionally close to is more difficult than saying no to complete strangers. Because of its wider social implication, the pressure exercised by people that are in some way close to us is hard to manage. So, as soon as you hear 'shots time!' you either flee the scene or stick with your NO. Say 'No, thanks' with a firm voice and with a smile.

And when you are struggling — because in certain situations we all do, no matter how driven we are — remember what makes you the most uncomfortable is often very effective. Personally, when I'm struggling with saying no to overeating and drinking, I try to remember that annoying feeling of *my favourite shirt* being too tight on my abdomen when I get unfit. This strategy works for me, but find what works for you.

91

6
RESISTANCE TO CHANGE

Since I was little, I was taught that the patience and foresight to see beyond the immediate and scan the far horizon is key to success. This is not surprising because my parents come from the farming culture that requires planning, patience and hard work to break the soil, plant the seeds, wait for the time to harvest the crops and pick the fruit. This was a concept that has been reinforced during my life through my experience as a kickboxing fighter, academic student, trainer and coach. Along the way I have met people who are incredibly successful in their career, in their relationships, in their physique, but I have yet to meet anyone who has achieved incredible success overnight. Success is a gradual evolution, a long series of small wins and tiny breakthroughs.

With this in mind, I will now put together the learnings of the previous five chapters, while introducing a tool that I believe is generally under-rated, though it is key in the quest of every successful person to get everything important done during their demanding day, including sticking to a fitness schedule and diet.

My clients sometimes invite me to their parties, black-tie dinners, champagne brunches and movie premiers. It is a privilege to see my clients shine and enjoy themselves in the company of their friends and colleagues, and for me to converse with other engaging and accomplished people. At some point in the conversation, due to the nature of my work, we talk about their fitness routines and diet. Usually these people say they are aiming for improvements, be it simply getting leaner or attaining measurable objectives, such as becoming faster and stronger.

Now here is the interesting part — overwhelmingly, these people say that they are unhappy with the results of past attempts at changing their fitness and eating regime. However, they are confident that if they were to start again tomorrow they would achieve the targets they set themselves, because this time they would try harder and stay committed. It is at this point that I can't help but ask:

● **Have you thought about and identified why you didn't achieve the desired results last time you tried? And if not, why do you think this time will be different?**

These two questions usually cause a mix of surprise and confusion, which might not be pleasant. After a few moments, the person I'm speaking with usually tries to get back in control by asserting that this time will be different, since they are very motivated. I have a good memory, and so remember faces and conversations. When I come across the same person again, I usually ask them if they got to where they wanted to with their fitness. Most of the time, the answer is 'no'.

Regardless of how often I experience this situation, I am still always surprised. What strikes me as unusual is the difference in approach that these people have to just about everything else, other than their fitness. These tend to be highly skilled and driven individuals who plan to the smallest detail when it comes to their careers, family affairs and personal development. Importantly, they tend to be aware of what holds them back and what helps them achieve their goals. They are also aware that long-term, durable results require planning, consistent effort and the capacity to tolerate temporary setbacks. Above all, they are aware of a universal rule:

Change triggers resistance

This is simply Newton's third law of motion restated. That law states that every action triggers an equal and opposite reaction. For example, every change in routine requires a change of habit, and the more intense in magnitude and more immediate in time the change is imposed, the stronger the resistance triggered. Whether you will achieve the change you want will depend on how you handle the resistance that will arise. A TV producer embarking on a project that has a set schedule will be aware that they will have to make changes to their working and rest routines, that their expectations will have to be adjusted and that there will be setbacks along the way. They will need to plan for how they will handle the setbacks, and be at peace with the fact that the results might take a while to materialise.

But interestingly, when it comes to their own diet and fitness goals, they don't tend to apply the same mindset. They are aware that the greater the change they aim for, the greater the resistance they will face. Nevertheless, when it comes to fitness and eating, they don't expect setbacks and they don't prepare for them. That's why they expect to shift to a whole new exercise and nutrition regime in a matter of days. That's why they fail to recognise the obstacles as part of the resistance to change, that might have held them back in the past during their previous attempts to reach their goals. From my conversations with them, the main reason they state is that they don't want fitness and eating to *feel like work*. Because their job is stressful and drains their mental energy, they are more likely to rely on inspiration in the moment and willpower to manage their fitness and diet, instead of planning like they do when they work.

But neither inspiration nor motivation stay consistently strong throughout the day, not to mention the week or month. How much you might wish to do something depends a lot on your available mind space. Furthermore, what you are inspired to achieve, and how motivated you are to apply yourself to get there, will clash with the various types of resistance to change. How that resistance to change in fitness and eating habits will manifest is unique to you. The most common types of resistance are:

1. Physiological resistance. The body itself mounts a great deal of physiological resistance to most attempts at fast or intense change. There is a state of homeostasis which is an optimal balance between energy consumed and energy expended — and it is something the body works quite hard to maintain. In other words, the body gets used to its current state, no matter how unfit or unhealthy, and any sudden or intense change will be resisted by this physiological habit. If you hit it with an intense exercise regime to rapidly gain muscle or lose fat, the body will fight hard to keep its previous patterns of energy consumption and expenditure, thus working against those changes. That is to say, your body will work hard against the results that you want to rapidly achieve. Following a rapid and intense change to types of activity you do and the way you eat, you might feel hungrier, prone to mood swings, physically tense and stiff.

2. Behavioural resistance. In chapter 1, we talked about how lack of mind space increases chances of reaching out for comfort/sugary foods and drinks. In chapter 2, we discussed that often people focus on exercising willpower to resist the impulse to reach out for those aides, rather than focusing on what triggers them to reach out in the first place. Imposing a sudden and intense change in physical activity or diet will often increase the behavioural/psychological resistance. Your mind, like your body, generally prefers to stick to the same routines and minimal change. Pushed into a new way of eating or getting to the gym early and often, you might find your mind asking '*Why am I here? Why am I doing this? What is the point?*'

3. Social pressure. In my career, I have seen clients expend precious willpower fighting social pressure to eat and drink at events, as we have seen in chapter 5. In addition to that, sometimes there is also a familial resistance that is particularly hard to work against because it is caused by a partner who behaves in a way that is in conflict with their fitness schedule and diet. I have always had the best results with clients who were supported by their partners, while we had poor results with clients with unsupportive partners.

4. Environmental and logistic resistance. Freezing cold, intense heat, humidity and heavy rain are some examples of environmental factors that could disrupt you from working out outside. For example, if you go to Singapore for a few days and you book a hotel without fitness facilities, you will find yourself fighting the humidity when running outdoors. Another example of logistic resistance is a gym that is very busy at lunchtime during your only available time to work out on weekdays.

5. Resistance from competition between goals and priorities. Let's assume that your goal is losing body fat. You want to lose some body fat, from a current weight of 80kg (with 22% body fat) to 75kg body weight (with 19% body fat). We will call that 'Goal A'. Let's also assume that nothing else mattered in your life and you are ready to do everything to reach Goal A. In this scenario, every decision you made during your day would be a binary choice that would bring you either closer to or farther away from Goal A:

Current situation: 80Kg ← DECISION → Goal A: 75Kg

For example, you are at the airport waiting for boarding. You only have a few minutes to buy something to eat and the only available food choices at the closest café are a tuna-mayo sandwich or salmon-greens-seeds box. This straightforward choice will take you either closer to or farther away from your goal of fat-loss: a tuna-mayo sandwich would get you farther away from Goal A, while the salmon-greens-seeds box would get you closer to it. It's quite simple and straightforward. The reality is that you have many goals and priorities in life, and so you will be forced to make decisions that get you closer to some goals while simultaneously pushing you farther away from others. Sometimes, those decisions will clash with your priorities.

The various conflicts between goals and priorities create confusion, increase stress and anxiety. This results in a loss of inspiration, motivation and persistence. For example, let's say that now you have two goals. Goal A is losing body fat. Goal B is to get a promotion this year. You also have priorities. These could be seeing your kids every night before they go to bed (priority 1) and spending more time with your partner (priority 2). It's Wednesday night and after a long day at work you are about to leave and go home to have a healthy dinner with your family, put the kids to bed, talk to your partner, go to bed early and get up the following morning fresh enough to work out first thing in the morning.

But just before you leave work, you are asked by important clients to join them to celebrate closing a very important deal with *a few drinks*. In that moment the choice is not binary anymore. Going to the bar would get you closer to your career goal (B) but at the same time farther from your fat-loss goal

(A) because you definitely won't be able to work out in the morning. You also would be deciding against your priorities 1 and 2. Another option is that you could just go to the bar for an hour and not drink alcohol (or drink only water while pretending it's a spirit with soda). This way you would satisfy the expectations of your clients (and get closer to Goal B), and limit empty calorie intake (advancing towards Goal A). Unless you miss out on the evening with clients, you will miss out on seeing your children and partner — so the decision to go to the event will clash with your family priorities.

Identifying your goals and priorities, and staying aware of the competing demands they place on you, is essential for preserving mind space. The greater your awareness of the clashes, the greater your capacity to make decisions in advance, rather than reacting to daily stressors impulsively.

● ● ●

I have seen that clients who are most successful in obtaining desirable results and maintaining them are those who are well-equipped to manage the various forms of resistance. Generally, it helps to just be aware that those resistances will come up. That by itself will help you plan ahead and handle them when they do pop up. However, awareness and some vague planning is not enough. You need a better, more specific tool, which I most imaginatively call 'forward planning'.

The structure of forward planning

1) Goal setting. The goal has to be clear.

2) Timeframe. The timeframe set to achieve the goal must be realistic.

3) Problems & solutions. Identify the factors which might disrupt you reaching your goal, and identify every possible solution, if it exists, for every single problem.

4) Action steps. Make a list of to-do's based on goals, problems and solutions.

5) Mechanisms of control. Measure, record and create micro-goals and long-term targets.

6) Accountability. Be accountable for every single action step.

It is quite intuitive. In the broadest terms, this is a way of moving from goal setting at the beginning to accountability at the end — and not the other way around. Curiously, when it comes to changing fitness and eating habits, people try to do it backwards. They try to be to be **accountable (6)** without being able to keep any **control (5)** over their **action steps (4),** **because they**'re not based on **solutions to problems (3)** that they have recognised. Due to an unrealistic **timeframe (2)** there is a sense of anxiety with sticking to a goal that is not **clear (1)**.

This makes it unsurprising that most fitness resolutions made at New Year are broken by February. The resolutionists don't lack for willpower, but given that the only bit of planning would usually be limited to buying food for a week and downloading a few workout routines, willpower does not last much beyond six weeks. What is lacking is serious consideration of what held them back last time, and a realistic assessment of what can be done about these factors.

It is true that a goal without a plan is only a wish, and that if you fail to plan, you plan to fail. But planning must start with goal setting and lead to accountability, and not vice-versa.

So, let's tackle this planning process logically and effectively:

1. Goal setting

Setting a clear goal is key, because the clearer the reason why you are trying to achieve that goal, the stronger the motivation is during tough times. Whether the target is running a half marathon or losing inches off your waist, try to clarify with yourself the reason why you are doing it: to look better for your next family beach holiday? To feel more confident when you speak in public for that presentation at work? To be as fit as a 30-year-old when you will be 70?

Once the goal is clearly defined, now increase clarity further by visualising the goal. Visualise yourself when the goal you are aiming for has been achieved. What would success mean to you? What would it mean for the people around you?

How do you feel about being successful in your pursuit? See how you feel when you visualise success. You might feel happy and joyful, however anxiety and numbness are not uncommon. And the latter happens when, although a goal is clearly defined, we discover we don't care much about hitting it.

Social pressure towards looking a certain way affects your choice of goal. Maybe what is motivating you could be aggressive advertising or social pressure, and in the end those aren't the forces that will sustain you when the going gets tough. Trying to achieve a goal that isn't personally important to you is a waste of time, consumes a lot of energy and would be a source of unnecessary anxiety. That's why through visualisation we can understand if we deeply care about achieving that goal. What are you doing this for? Is it for aesthetic reasons (for yourself or for a partner/friends)? Is it for health reasons? Is it so you are able to play with the kids, walk to work, not feel out of breath after a specific activity? The more specific the visualisation, the more authentic the feelings you might experience when you try to visualise yourself as successful in your pursuit. It is this authenticity of experience and intimacy with how you feel about achieving your goals that will help you stay motivated when the tough times come — which of course, they always do.

'I want to lose 6kg of body fat for my next family holiday. I can see myself on the beach, with a narrower waist, tighter abdomen, toned arms. I am smiling and enjoying being able to play beach games with my kids and taking photos with my partner. I look forward to start!'

2. Timeframe

Whatever the goal you wish to achieve, be specific about when you would like to get there. Define a realistic timeframe. The goal needs to be achievable by a specific date, not too close and not too far. I always ask my clients: '*What's the next date in the calendar*' to consistently keep clear in their mind, and mine, what we are aiming to achieve and by when. Our brain works better with a clear timeframe — it keeps motivation and inspiration high. But the date that you have set in your calendar to achieve your goal must be realistic, because your motivation and capacity to stay strong with your decisions will be effected by how close or far you perceive that date to be. If the date feels too far out then it will be easy to relax a bit too much. If the date feels too close, then anxiety would rise, negative inner dialogue would kick in, mind space reduce, and procrastination and wrong food choices are more likely to happen. Overall, your perception of the gap between what you have, what you want, and the effort that you forecast you will need to put in, will trigger stress as either excitement or anxiety. When this stress is enough to keep you going then it's positive excitement, if the stress is too much then anxiety kicks in, and you will more likely feel overwhelmed and give up.

Now, check your calendar and look for dates to aim for. This could be a public talk, a job interview, an important dinner or a sport competition like a run for charity, or a school mates' reunion to play a sport. It doesn't need to be focused on aesthetics or performance, it could be purely focused on the way you want to feel. Having a list of dates to aim for makes it easier for your mind to stick to them. Once you have a clear and visualised goal in mind, and you know you are fully committed to achieving it, set your timeframe. Let's assume that you have a family holiday *in three months' time*. That's your timeframe. If you aim for a massive change too fast, you will fight against a whole collection of strong resistances. Little changes within a realistic timeframe feel easier, ingrain deeper into daily life, and last longer.

3. Problems & solutions

By definition, your goal is a state that you are not in right now. Identify and write down a list of factors that might hamper your progress from your current state towards your desired end state (goal). In my experience of working with top performers with busy lives, apart from common disruptive factors — such as an overcrowded mind space, lack of routine, many social events, cravings for sugary comfort foods and lack of quality sleep — there are other factors which are more specific to every individual. Ideally, you would identify every single problem that is personal to you, and if possible, a solution to each and every one.

4. Action steps

Once you are clear about your goal, about when you would like to get there, and what might hinder you along the way, take time to identify actions that need to be taken.

For example, if your colleagues at work bring everyday food rich in added sugar like cupcakes and cakes that you struggle to avoid eating (**problem**), you want to bring with you sweet snacks without any added sugar for example some fresh fruit (**solution**). Once you identified the solution the action steps would be:

Action step 1: update your weekly online food-shopping list to bring fruit with you from home.

Action step 2: get up earlier to have the time to buy fruit on the way to work.

5. Mechanisms of control

Mechanisms of control are tools that make you aware of which stage of your plan you are at. Knowing at any time if you are on target or not is important to keep motivation high and to be able to make changes, whenever necessary, to increase the chances of hitting your goal. Mechanisms of control don't rely on feelings.

One of the mistakes that I have noticed people make is to rely on their feelings to judge whether they are achieving results or not. I'm sure you check your bank account, business account and your investment stocks rather than think: *'I feel like I am making/losing money'*. Feelings change during the day, feelings are not objective and so feelings are misleading. If you don't measure, you don't know what's happening, and if you don't know what's happening you cannot correct it.

Mechanisms of control are expressed by numbers like circumference of waist in centimetres, body weight in kilograms, amount of weekly running in kilometres, amount of weekly training sessions, weekly nutritional calorie deficit — just to mention a few. When we see numbers on paper then we know what's happening and whether you are on target or not. When you are not on target, then you can make corrections to your fitness and diet plan, maintaining control over the process and increasing your chances of success. And when you are on target and you see positive results with real numbers on paper, then you feel even more inspired and motivated to see more results. It has a powerful effect on your perception of the effort it takes to work out and/or eat a certain way. This can be visualised by the equation:

Value Perception = Reward – Pain

In this equation, reward is the outcome one desires in a given context (things we want to have, to do, or to be) and pain is the price, time and effort involved. When you see results, the reward increases and the perception of pain decreases. And so your perception towards a task changes. That's why at some point we start to perceive something that in the past was painful as easy to do, exciting and rewarding. Examples of other rewards that change the perception of pain could be: increasing the distance of your run every week, or improving your personal best with squats or deadlifts every week. Seeing results on paper will help you focus and increase your confidence in the plan. In my experience, the most effective mechanisms of control are:

1. Measure and record. Keeping track of biometrics,

sessions and meals is incredibly effective to keep motivation high. When you track and see results on paper, you feel much more motivated and inspired to keep going.

> ▶ **Biometrics:** body weight, centimetres of waist/arms/legs, body fat percentage. Measure and record on a weekly basis. Having this data to look back on will dramatically alter how in control you feel about what is going on with you and your body.

> ▶ **Number and type of sessions per week:** with notes about performance (weights, mileage for running/swimming).

> ▶ **Food diary:** make a record of meal calories with a smartphone app. You will have an instant breakdown of calories, macronutrients and micronutrients.

2. Split long-term macro-goals into short-term micro-goals. Setting up shorter-term targets to your longer-term goals.

> ▶ If your macro-goal is losing 6kg of body fat in three months, then your micro-goals would be losing 2kg per month, so 500 grams per week. This way, if you are not on target, you can decide to change something with your workout and/or your diet. If you are on target, your motivation will feed on your short-terms achievements, pushing you forward.

3. Be in credit with your workouts. It is best to stay slightly ahead of your target, rather than feel that you need to catch up.

▶ For example, if you have planned to do two resistance training sessions per week (Monday/Thursday), one circuit conditioning class (Tuesday) and one cardio session (Saturday), that's four sessions per week, 16 sessions per month and 48 sessions over the three months' timeframe you have before your holiday to lose 6kg of body fat. As your weekly target is four sessions, in case you would do only two sessions in the first week, you then need to make up for it with six sessions the following week to be on target.

Your expectation for yourself will be to make up for it the next week — which some people find disheartening. So, in the first week you should try to do five sessions, then you will be one session ahead. Knowing that you are in credit, that you are ahead, will increase your motivation and keep you stronger. I call it momentum, many people call it 'in the zone'. Being in credit is very motivating and calming, because when you miss a few training sessions due to a bad week at work or illness, knowing that you are still on target because you did very well the weeks before, makes you feel like you are carrying on something you were good at, rather than starting again from square one. The key is to be as healthy as you can now, so that if something ever happens, you're in a better position to deal with it properly, whatever it may be. Knowing you're ahead increases your sense of control and it keeps motivation and momentum high.

6. Accountability

Now you've set a clear goal within a realistic timeframe, recognised possible problems and found solutions to them, you have a list of action steps and mechanisms of control. It's time to think about and implement the ways in which you can be held accountable. I do believe that accountability has a genetic component, it's mainly a natural skill. I've noticed over the years that most successful individuals are accountable for what they plan, no matter what. These individuals somehow do what they say they would do, including working out and eating a certain way, unless very rare and unfortunate events occur. They don't act according to feelings or inner dialogue, but instead according to plan. I still don't know whether this skill is genetic or if it can be learnt and developed further. There are strategies that people with a low accountability skill can rely on to keep consistency with a plan. For example, at a simple level, booking several classes in advance and paying for them increases the chances that people will attend them. Similarly so, booking a training course with a personal trainer, or pairing up with a reliable colleague or friend who is accountable and rarely cancels. Personally, my accountability mainly feeds off my diary management. Whenever I don't feel like training and I struggle to motivate myself, I check my diary and often just seeing that I won't have time to work out for the next one or two days will motivate me into doing it.

• • •

Beginning a radical change in the way you manage your physical activity and eating habits — with a commitment to a new exercise regime and a new diet — and then expending precious willpower to stick with it 'no matter what' is putting accountability before all the other stages. Unfortunately, that is often how people, no matter how smart they are, approach fitness and eating. It is extremely hard if not impossible to be **accountable (6)** without using **mechanisms of control (5)** over **action steps (4)** that are not based on recognised **solutions to problems (3)**. Due to an unrealistic **timeframe (2)** there would be a sense of anxiety with sticking to a goal that is not **clear (1)**. Going from 6 to 1 would increase the various forms of resistance even more, requiring more effort, more mind space and more time. Conversely, when you follow the way of planning in the right order, from 1 to 6, you dramatically increase your odds of achieving results, while feeling in control of your life, motivated, strengthening your self-esteem and enjoying a priceless sense of achievement that will push you even further towards unexpected, positive and long-lasting results.

Having a solid plan in place provides sharp focus and excitement, while preventing ambiguity, doubts, anxiety and the various form of resistance. While a plan can be revisited and modified, the absence of a plan excludes feedback, control, effective use of time, progressions and long-lasting results. Conversely, if you see from your record that you are not improving, you are more likely to understand why by asking a professional or an experienced friend. Only when you measure and record what's happening will you be able to correct the action steps.

If you cannot measure it, you cannot correct it. And only

what gets measured gets managed. You cannot rely only on how you feel to determine that a plan is working or not. Feelings can be misleading. Knowing what's happening and knowing what to do is highly motivating. And when you are able to measure results, whenever you have achieved results, you then feel in the zone, and you feel inspired and motivated.

7
SOLUTIONS TO COMMON PROBLEMS

Now let's see my suggested solutions, and action steps, to the ten most common problems that I've found busy individuals face on their daily quest to get (and stay) fit while juggling between priorities and goals.

Problem 1

You don't have a fitness plan, so you go to the gym and you do some exercises or classes according to how you feel. When you don't give a consistent stimulus to your body, it will put up even more resistance to change in the form of fatigue, muscle and joint pain (physiological resistance). When you don't know what to do fitness-wise, your motivation will fade during those days when your mind space is overcrowded (behavioural/psychological resistance).

Solution: Select the right fitness plan with the type of workouts that work for you (for example cardio based, metabolic conditioning, resistance training, boxing, etc.) and make a consistent weekly schedule.

Action step: Research (the web, specific books, or ask a professional at your local gym) and find the most highly recommended fitness plans for your weight loss goal. Once you have decided which type of fitness plan suits you best, write down your weekly schedule. For example: Two resistance training sessions per week (Monday/Thursday), one circuit conditioning class (Tuesday) and one cardio session (Saturday). Write down your gym workouts. Having a written plan makes it easier to change or adapt a few exercises in a fully packed gym, while saving mental space and time.

Problem 2

Your job makes you mentally too tired to train in the evening (psychological resistance).

Solution: Work out first thing in the morning.

Action step: Streamline the 'wake up and go training' process by relying on consistent night routines: prepare your training kit so its ready for the morning, have a training routine written down (so you know what to do), go to bed early. Improve your quality of sleep with the strategies we have seen in chapter 3.

Problem 3

There are often conflicts between your work schedule, family schedule and fitness schedule. Your work diary gets filled with meetings booked by your boss/co-workers/assistant. Events that involve family and friends feel like they're coming out of nowhere and last minute (resistance triggered by competition between goals and priorities).

Solution: Keep every work, social, family event and workout in your electronic calendar.

Action step: Block slots for training in your work electronic diary by every Friday for the following week. Ask your partner, relatives and friends to send you invitations by email that automatically go into your calendar for every event you agreed to attend (parties, family reunions etc.)

Problem 4

You eat according to how you feel in the moment. When you don't give a consistent stimulus for your body, it will put up even more resistance to change in the form of unjustified intense hunger and cravings for comfort food like biscuits and crisps (physiological resistance).

Solution: Find the right diet for you, try to eat at the same few places and use a mental pathway (as seen in chapter 2) to put a meal together, wherever you are and in every situation.

Action step: Research the web, or ask a professional, for the most advisable diet for your weight loss goal. Once you have decided which type of diet suits you, write down your weekly meal plan, including snacks. Remember that a diet, as way of living, must support your lifestyle and keep you healthy and productive without triggering stress and anxiety.

Problem 5

You are too tired after work to go shopping and cook. This

often makes you fall back onto packaged convenience food (behavioural resistance, environmental resistance).

Solution: Order your fresh and healthy food online with a weekly delivery. Once the list is made, you will only need to update it whenever you need to. Online shopping saves you time that you would otherwise spend after work.

Action step: Make the list according to your diet plan and weekly meal plan.

Problem 6

During the week you crave sugar at work, mainly between 3pm and 4pm, and often when you are working on a boring task while sitting in a chair for hours (physiological resistance, behavioural/psychological resistance).

Solution: Bring healthy snacks to work and get rid of the unhealthy food in your desk drawers. Stay seated as little as possible, as spending too many hours in a chair triggers cravings for sugary foods.

Action step: On your food shopping list, include healthy snacks to bring to work during the week. Stand up often, keep moving and be mobile.

Problem 7

One hour after dinner, no matter what and how much you eat, you often crave something with sugar and you often give in (behavioural/psychological resistance, environmental resistance).

Solution: Use the WWH technique as seen in chapter 4, to understand whether your sugar craving is triggered by stress, anxiety, boredom or any other emotion.

Action step: Eliminate from the kitchen cupboards and drawers anything containing sugar. Have herbal tea 30 minutes after dinner. Brush your teeth after you have finished your tea. Go to bed by 10pm to avoid the 10–11pm craving window.

Problem 8

Looking at your diary for the next three months, you can see that you have five friends' birthday parties and three work events to attend. You know now that you will need to manage unhealthy served food and lots of pressure to drink (social pressure, environmental resistance, competition between goals and priorities).

Solution: Mentally prepare yourself and decide how much you want to drink before every single social event.

Action step: Use the strategies we covered in chapter 5.

117

Problem 9

Looking at your diary, you have an old friend coming to town for a weekend. Every time you see him, somehow you cannot say 'no thanks' to him when he insists you drink alcohol (social pressure, environmental resistance, competition between goals and priorities).

Solution: He drinks a lot, especially at night, hence this time round you will try to see him during the day for brunch instead.

Action step: Send your friend a text to put brunch in the calendar.

Problem 10

Your partner appears to not be supportive of you with regards to your fitness and diet plan (behavioural/psychological resistance).

This happens very often for various reasons. The most common is lack of clarity and miscommunication. (My experience is that having a collaborative partner makes the journey towards the goal much easier, while having a disruptive partner slows the process down).

Solution: Talk to your partner: explain your goal, your reasons and ask for more support.

Action step: Clarity in your own head will help to find the best way to explain your purpose to your partner. Answer these questions in order to get ready for that difficult conversation. Does your partner know how important the goal is to you? Have you been consistent with your actions or did you send confusing signals? Could your partner be confused by your attempt to change? How could the achievement of your goal change your relationship with your partner?

CONCLUSION

The fast pace of modern life puts a lot of pressure on the minds and bodies of individuals who want to be good at their jobs, be present for their families and friends, and be reasonably fit. The daily marathon through deadlines, commutes, responsibilities, chores and events can increase overall stress and anxiety, hamper the quality of sleep, lead to procrastination and cravings for comfort food.

During my 20+ years' experience as personal trainer and daily productivity coach for busy and successful people who want to have it all, I had to find tools and strategies to reduce the detrimental effect that their demanding lifestyles had on their fitness schedule, diet and energy levels.

How can you prevent willpower from succumbing to decision-fatigue during the day? How can you ensure that your precious little available time to work out doesn't go wasted because of a drop in motivation? How do you make yourself get up on a cold morning to go for a run? How do you stay committed to going to the gym after a long day at work? How can you reduce the chances of drinking and eating too much at a friend's party or work event? How can you avoid reaching for comfort food when under pressure? How can you increase the quality of your sleep during those scarce available hours?

I found that the key is keeping mentally, emotionally and physically strong during your hectic day. In order to do this:

1. Keep available mind space to reduce procrastination and cravings for comfort food

- Keep your mind de-cluttered
- Make your environment work for you, not against you
- Be in control of your diary

2. Reduce decision fatigue to save willpower

- Create and rely on well-established morning, night-time and weekend routines
- Break those unhealthy routines that are holding you back

3. Get quality sleep to keep sound in mind and body

- Use conscious breathing techniques
- Focus on mindfulness and compartmentalization
- Optimise your sleeping environment

4. Nurture your digestive system to be more resilient to illness

- Feed your gut's good microbiome, starve your gut's harmful microbiome
- Identify and avoid foods which you are intolerant and sensitive to, if any
- Get a grip on your emotional eating by using the WWH technique

5. Be ready for every social event to avoid over-eating and over-drinking

- Plan what and how much you will eat and drink
- Use specific strategies to handle social pressure and stick to the plan

6. Use forward planning to push you towards your goals (with less Resistance).

- Move from goal-setting to accountability, not vice-versa
- Set a realistic time-frame
- Identify problems and find solutions to each of them
- Make a list of action steps and be accountable
- Maintain control by measuring, recording and creating micro-goals and long-term targets

Remember that when you make small positive changes, they will only trigger a little resistance, so these new healthy habits are more likely to become engrained into your everyday life with little effort and very powerful results.

I hope that this book has given you useful tools that you have already started to implement little by little into your busy day.

Giac

SHORT WORKOUTS

With STRONG I wanted to give you effective tools to power your existing fitness schedule, which means doing that workout you have planned despite your busy schedule, while avoiding procrastination and wasting precious time. And it also means keeping inspired enough to do a workout whenever you have available time due to a last-minute opening in your diary. Very often these last-minute workouts need to be short in order to fit into a small time slot.

Short workouts make it easier to keep you ahead of your monthly workout target. As we said in chapter 6, being *in credit and not in debit* with your workouts is key to offset those days/weeks when you will be unable to exercise due to your work and family schedule, or illness. Because, of course, those days / weeks will happen.

There are plenty of great books, websites and smartphone apps with 15—40 minute long workouts that can be done anywhere, with or without equipment. Nevertheless, I want to give you my favourites that my clients and myself use to keep up momentum. The following short workouts all

◗ Require little mind space
◗ Maximise calorie burn and increase metabolic rate
   during and after the workout, from two hours to
   24 hours after your workout (depending on intensity
   and duration).
◗ Increase your capacity for high-intensity exercise
◗ Make you move under various planes or work hence
   keeping your body functional and balanced

Remember: Always start with a warm-up that can be a mix of stretching, flexibility drills, callisthenics or a few minutes on a cardio-vascular machine. Get your joints and muscles warm and your heart rate slightly up. During the session remember to keep your heart rate right for your medical history and training background. After the session I always suggest to cool down while lying on the floor for a few minutes doing some stretching and breathing.

1) THE BASICS (20–40 minutes)

I call them The Basics because these routines are made of a combination of 6 basic movements: squatting, bending, lunging, pushing, pulling, and twisting. The exercises are high compound that means they involve multiple muscles and joints during the execution. High compound exercises not only burn lot of calories but they also stimulate the production of good hormones responsible for keeping muscle tissue and getting good quality sleep. The equipment necessary can be free weights, machines or just your body weight. The exercises are organised in pairs, for example:

3 sets x 10 reps, 30 seconds Rest Period (RP)
A1 Squatting exercise
A2 Pulling exercise

3x10, 30sec RP
B1 Bending
B2 Pushing exercise

3x10, 30sec RP
C1 Lunging exercise
C2 Twisting exercise

Method of execution:

▶ Do A1 for 10 repetitions then rest for 30 seconds
▶ Do A2 for 10 repetitions and rest for 30 seconds
▶ Do A1+A2 again 2 more times, while resting for 30 seconds after every set.
▶ Once you have completed (A1+A2)x3, use the same method with the next couple of exercises B1 and B2. Therefore execute (B1+B2)x3 while resting for 30 seconds after every set.
▶ Once you have done (B1+B2)x3, use the same method with the last couple of exercises C1 and C2.

The rest period between the exercises can differ between 15 seconds, 30 seconds, 45 seconds and 60 seconds according with the intensity you want to give to your session, the weight you lift and the time you have available. I find working out with 10 repetitions as ideal to keep the right balance between building muscular strength and endurance, and also to keep the risk of injury low. If you only have weights available that are *slightly too heavy* to be able to finish 10 reps, use a range between 6-8 reps instead. At the opposite, in case you only have weights that are *slightly too light* that enables you to comfortably do more than 10 reps, use a range between 12-15 reps.

Considering both effectiveness and safety, my favourite basic exercises to build a short workout are (not in order of preference):

A1 Squatting exercises:
▶ Squats
▶ Barbell back squat
▶ Single dumbbell squat
▶ Landmine squats
▶ Jumping squat
▶ Box jump

A2 Pulling exercises:
▶ Pull-ups/chin-ups on a bar or gymnastic rings
▶ Lat-machine pull down (with various grips)
▶ Bent over row with barbell or dumbbells
▶ Single arm bent over row with dumbbell (on a bench)
▶ Renegade row with 2 dumbbells/kettle-bells

❯ Seated or standing pulley row (low or medium start)

❯ Inverted row with TRX or gymnastic rings

❯ Landmine bent over row

B1 Bending exercises:

❯ Deadlifts with barbell or dumbbells or kettle-bells

❯ Deadlifts with dumbbells on an upside down BOSU ball

❯ Single leg deadlifts with/without dumbbell or kettle-bell

❯ Single leg deadlifts on an upside down BOSU ball

❯ Hyperextensions at the inclined or horizontal hyperextension machine, with/without a weight

B2 Pushing exercises:

❯ Press-ups with/without 2 dumbbells or 2 kettle-bells or parallettes or gymnastic rings

❯ Horizontal or inclined bench press with barbell or dumbbells

❯ Floor presses with dumbbells

❯ Dips at the parallel bars or with gymnastic rings

❯ Standing or sitting shoulder presses with barbell or dumbbells or kettle-bells

C1 Lunging exercises:

❯ Lunges with/without dumbbells or kettle-bells

❯ Lunges on a upside down BOSU ball

❯ Walking lunges with/without dumbbells or kettle-bells

❯ Back lunges with/without dumbbells or kettle-bells

❯ Back lunges on an upside down BOSU ball

❱ Step up on a box with/without dumbbells or kettle-bells

C2 Twisting exercise:
❱ Cable twist (horizontal or low-to-high or high-to-low)
❱ Wood chop with dumbbell or medicine ball
❱ Cable archer row
❱ Single arm cable chest press (with rotation)
❱ Landmine twist

Note: when you put a workout together I advise to keep your sessions as contained as possible which means staying in the same meter square and/or using pieces of equipment that are close to each other, especially in busy gyms. Considering all the above, let's see an example (note that the choice of weights is purely illustrative):

THE BASICS, example 1

Warm-up

3 sets x 10 reps, 30 seconds Rest Period (RP)
A1 Squat barbell @40kg
A2 Renegade rows dumbbells @10kg

3x10, 30sec RP
B1 Deadlifts barbell @50kg
B2 Dumbbells floor press @14kg

3x10, 30sec RP
C1 Lunges with dumbbells @4kg each
C2 Horizontal cable twist @15kg

Cool down

Once you have a written plan it will be easy to change a few exercises in case the gym is too busy or the equipment is scarce. For example in case the squat rack was busy or unavailable, then grab a bench and a few dumbbells and do:

THE BASICS, example 2

Warm-up

3 sets x 10 reps, 30 seconds Rest Period (RP)
A1 Single dumbbell squat @14kg
A2 Single arm bent over row with dumbbell @18kg

3x10, 30sec RP
B1 Deadlifts dumbbells @20kg
B2 Chest press dumbbells @16kg

3x10, 30sec RP
C1 Step ups on box (use the bench as a box)
C2 Wood chop with dumbbell @6kg

Cool down

If you want to be even more time effective you can cut your rest period while adding a few low compound exercises that target a specific area or muscle group like your glutes or abs. This is possible with adding a third exercise to each pair of exercises. Like the following example:

THE BASICS, example 3

Warm-up

3x, 15 seconds Rest Period (RP)
A1 Landmine squat 10 reps @10kg
A2 Landmine bent over row 10 reps @15kg
A3 Glutes fire hydrants 20 reps (each side)

3x, 15sec RP
B1 Single leg deadlifts on an upside down BOSU ball
B2 Standing shoulder press with dumbbells
10 reps @10Kg
B3 Plank 30sec

3x, 15sec RP
C1 Back lunges on an upside down BOSU ball 10 reps
C2 Landmine twist 20 reps
C3 Glute bridge 20 reps

Cool down

2) THE DOWNHILL 5-4-3-2-1 (Less than 20 minutes)

This is a circuit of 4 high compound exercises to be completed using two dumbbells. The fact that the repetitions decrease after each individual set keeps you motivated because you can foresee the *finish line*. The exercises are:

A1 Deadlifts with dumbbells

A2 Dumbbells squats + shoulder press

A3 Standing dumbbells row

A4 Press-ups on dumbbells

Method of execution:

▶ Grab two dumbbells and do A1+A2+A3+A4 for 5 repetitions each exercise without resting.

▶ Do A1+A2+A3+A4 again for 4 repetitions each exercise without resting.

▶ Do A1+A2+A3+A4 for 3 repetitions each without resting.

▶ Do A1+A2+A3+A4 for 2 repetitions each without resting.

▶ Do A1+A2+A3+A4 for 1 repetition without resting.

▶ Finally rest for 1 minute.

▶ Repeat again all the above for 2 more sets.

For an easier version do the squat without shoulder pressing. And/or do press-ups with your hands on the floor instead of using the dumbbells. The Downhill circuit can be done easily at home or in any hotel gym.

3) SPRINTING (Less than 15 minutes)

▶ **Sprinting between two points**. Whenever you want to sprint in the park, in a safe street, in a football/basketball court or on the beach: select a point A, walk for 30 wide long steps to point B. Use anything visible like a bottle or your jacket to mark point B. Sprint from point A to point B. Walk back to point A. As soon as you have reached point A turn around quick and sprint to point B again. Repeat 10 times. Rest for 1 minute. Repeat the 10 sprints for 2 more sets keeping 1 minute rests in between the sets.

- 3 sets x (10 sprints x 30 meters between A and B).
- Walk back to A after you sprint to B.
- 1 minute of rest in between the 3 sets.

(You can sprint also on 45 or 60 meters and use 90secs or 120secs rest period)

▶ **Treadmill push sprints.** On a treadmill (turned off), grab the bar in front of you (normally where the sensors are to check your heart rate), lean forward and start moving the tape by pushing with your legs. As soon as you take decent speed (running) start counting 30 steps. After that stop for 10 seconds. Repeat 4 more times. Take 1 minute of rest. Repeat the above routine for 2 more sets.

- 3 sets x (5 sprints x 30 steps).
- 10 seconds of rest in between the sprints.

• 1 minute of rest in between the 3 sets.

(You can increase the number of sets to 4 or 5, and the steps up to 100)

4) JUMP ROPE (Less than 15 minutes)

Not only does jump rope have many benefits like improving coordination, footwork and sense of rhythm, it is also very time effective if you consider that *10 minutes skipping medium pace equals 20 minutes running medium pace.*

Do 3 rounds x 2 minutes. Skip fast at 80-90% of your max speed for 10 seconds, and then skip at 30-40% of your max speed for 10 seconds. Keep alternating speed every 10 seconds for the whole 2 minutes round. Rest for 1 minute after the first round. Repeat for at least 2 more rounds.

• 3 x 2 minutes rounds.
• Skip fast at 80-90% of your max speed for 10 seconds, and then skip at 30-40% of your max speed for 10 seconds.
• Keep alternating the two speeds for 2 minutes.
• 1 minute of rest in between the rounds.

(You can either increase the number of rounds to 4 or 5, or the length to 3 minutes)

ABOUT THE AUTHOR

My name is Giac Farci. I am in my forties, and for more than 20 years I've been advising top performers in London, New York and Los Angeles on physical training, nutrition and improving their quality of life.

Through conversations between our training sessions at the gym, I have observed, learnt and gained valuable insights into the lives of my clients. Over the years, I have shared emotional, difficult and uplifting moments with them: career struggles, new business ventures, family crises, break-ups, new love stories and new-born babies. Through these encounters and my own personal experiences, I've gained a better understanding of the needs of highly successful people, and have developed new and effective strategies to help these top performers pursue their perfect balance in life.

Born in Sardinia with a form of anaemia called G6PD-deficiency or favism, I am intimately familiar with the challenge of a balanced life. Favism is a form of anaemia that protects against malaria, which is beneficial. The downside is that people with G6PD-deficiency have fewer and smaller red blood cells. Their capacity to carry oxygen is reduced, causing episodes of intense fatigue whenever there is an imbalance of physical activity and resting time.

Furthermore, people with G6PD-deficiency are also strongly allergic to the legume broad beans. Consumption of even a small amount of broad beans could lead to the breakdown of red blood cells, multiple organ failure, and eventual death if left without immediate medical treatment.

In addition, I am also intolerant to all other legumes like black beans, peas, chickpeas, lentils and peanuts. In order to avoid broad beans and legumes, I have learnt from an early age to check food labels and to enquire about the ingredients of the food that was given to me on school outings and at friends' parties. I also had to learn to continually manage my energy levels while attending school and playing sports, to prevent debilitating fatigue. This lifelong challenge forced me to educate myself about food, training and recovery time, which in turn shaped my approach to life and eventually my career.

I was 16 when I fell in love with kickboxing. After a few years, I had achieved my black belt and won trophies at the regional and national level. Soon enough, life became complicated from trying to juggle school, friends and sports. I had to find ways to reach and maintain the highest possible level of physical and mental energy to complete all the critical activities during a busy day. Every day was like walking across a tightrope while juggling multiple balls in the air. Learning how to maintain both the highest level of physical and mental fitness allowed me to continue my life as a top athlete while living with this G6PD-deficiency.

Competing at the highest level required me to reach a level of fitness that, due to my G6PD-deficiency, was really difficult to maintain. When I finished high school, I had stopped competing at the European level and I decided to pursue a degree in Sport and Exercise Science to expand my knowledge and understanding of physiology, psychology, neurophysiology, biomechanics, biochemistry, anatomy, biokinetics and immunology.

While pursuing my degree, I was afforded a life-changing experience working as a physical education teacher in a retirement home in a little town in the middle of Sardinia. This job influenced my approach as a personal trainer more than coaching classes at my kickboxing gym for children, adults, and pro-fighters, or working as the strength and conditioning trainer of the youth squad of a professional football team.

I still remember my first day at the retirement home. I was introduced to about 20 women and men with an average age of 84. They initially showed a mix of curiosity and suspicion, which wasn't surprising to me because I knew most of them had been farmers and had never had a physical education teacher before. When a woman in her late 70s, who at the time was still getting up at 5am to pick potatoes and tomatoes from her allocated land, challenged me to an arm-wrestle and I couldn't win, I knew I had landed in a very interesting place where I would learn a lot.

The daily quest of these elderly people was not about aesthetics or performance, nor only about living as long as possible. Their aim was to have a pain-free body to enjoy long walks in the countryside, and it was just as important for them to have a functioning mind to enjoy the visits of their dear ones.

It was this different angle on healthy living that made me look even deeper into the benefits of fitness in supporting a long and rewarding life. Today, according to a study made by National Geographic, Sardinia is still among one of the six areas (called 'blue zones') on the planet, with the highest percentage of ultra-centenaries. The other areas are Okinawa in Japan, Loma Linda in California, The Nicoya Peninsula in Costa Rica, and the Greek island Ikaria. The six 'blue zones' have many traits in common like a diet rich in vegetables and fish, and low on meat, refined sugar and refined flours. These ultra-centenaries still manage to keep a mobile body and a sharp mind to sustain an active lifestyle. They still cultivate vegetables in their gardens, they look after their big families (some of them having up to 25 grandchildren) and they enjoy their friends' company.

Inspired by the deep connection between mind, body and one's ability to live a fulfilling life with many goals and priorities, I decided to leverage my degree to pursue a career as a full-time personal trainer and coach. Once I obtained my Sport and Exercise Science degree, I moved to Rome to work for a commercial chain corporate gym.

The first weeks in the Eternal City were hectic with me trying to adapt to new everyday life dynamics in a new reality. Especially since work immediately became very busy with trying to build a new client base, as I had high weekly and monthly targets to hit for selling and delivering personal training sessions. Days were very long, overall 14 hours a day, and time to work out was scarce. Whenever I had just 30 minutes free to work out my thoughts were saying: 'If you cannot do a 60 to 90-minute-long session then don't bother. Train properly or don't.'

Although I was not competing anymore, I still had the sport-competitor mentality, therefore for me it was still a matter of 'training hard or going home'. Without realising it I started to reduce my workouts to those moments when I had more than one hour free, and this way I struggled for many months. During those months I was eating way more than necessary and my sleep was poor in quality, leading to less energy levels and an accumulation of body fat. At some point, after about one year, in a desperate attempt to change the loop I was stuck in I started to do short 20—30 minute sessions, every day. In a few weeks I felt my body getting leaner and strong again, my hunger diminishing, my sleep improving, my energy raising and my mind getting clearer. A bit of training every day was better than nothing. For a busy professional like me, a bit of training every day was better than a long session once in a while. This new mindset helped me to support my new lifestyle of early rises and late hours.

When everything in Rome was going well, things suddenly changed. I'd lost all my savings in a business venture. I was 30 years old and totally skint. After a few days spent on a friend's couch, I decided to get up and fight back.

I needed a new challenge, and so despite never having studied English, I moved to London. I'll spare you the details of my struggle with the language, with the weather, with the food — especially on a very low budget. In two years' time I became very busy again and after that I opened my own PT studio with a few business partners.

In the City of London I became specialised in training individuals with a particular lifestyle — those with highly

139

demanding jobs, tight family schedules and active social lives, such as investment bankers, corporate lawyers, movie producers and owners of companies. They all have a common goal in life, which is to find a perfect balance in their lives — professionally, emotionally and physically — allowing them to be good at their jobs, to be present for their families and friends, and to be reasonably fit.

Their daily challenge is to optimize their time, and their mental and physical energy to complete their daily marathon through many deadlines, commutes, responsibilities and chores. Their success rides on their ability to juggle the balls in the air while balancing as they walk across the tightrope. Although they don't have a lot of time, these top performers are driven, organized and accountable to their goals. They work to give their physical activity and correct eating habits the necessary time and attention. But due to their particular lifestyles, they tend to struggle when work gets too intense. They suffer from low energy due to lack of sleep or jet lag. An intense family schedule complicates things further with last minute emergencies, or there are simply just too many social events where they inevitably get bombarded with alcohol and unhealthy foods.

As soon as I started working with this particular type of client, I quickly realised that although I had an extensive martial arts and sports background, knew all the exercises, had tried all the diets and could recite all the motivational quotes, it was not enough. My old approach that had always worked in the past was not effective with these world-class performers. Just as when I worked with the elderly, I knew it was time to refocus, to study something new like life coaching, to change my old approach to make a real positive impact by tailoring programs to their individual lifestyles through unique strategies. These extremely busy and successful CEOs, bankers, lawyers, politicians, actors, movie producers and writers are all driven, motivated and inspiring individuals. I have learnt a lot from them: a positive mindset, continuous effort to improve, intense drive, planning skills and accountability — just to mention a few.

But make no mistake, when I talk about busy and successful people I don't refer to position in the social ladder or money. In fact, one of the best clients I have ever had, and in my opinion one of the most successful, was a single mum who was juggling between two part-time jobs and a son with a disability. She has got in touch and started working with me, with the main goal of getting physically stronger to be able move her son better, like bathing him, dressing him, and taking him in and out of the pram. Not only she has reached and maintained her main goal, but she has also improved her overall energy levels to sometimes feel like seeing a few friends after a very busy day.

Through my experience working with successful and busy people, not only did I get better at my work, but my whole life improved by learning from them. At the same time, I was able to make a positive impact on my clients' lives by providing them with unique tools and solutions to stay on top of their game.

My daily job is helping my clients to stay physically, mentally and emotionally strong so they can achieve everything without compromising their extremely busy lifestyle.

Giac

NOTES

Targeting Procrastination Using Psychological Treatments: A Systematic Review and Meta-Analysis. Alexander Rozental, Sophie Bennett, David Forsström, David D. Ebert, Roz Shafran, Gerhard Andersson and Per Carlbring. Front. Psychol. 2018.

Pressed for time? Goal conflict shapes how time is perceived, spent, and valued. J Etkin, I Evangelidis, J Aaker. Journal of Marketing Research, 2015

Emotional influences on food choice: Sensory, physiological and psychological pathways. Edward Leigh Gibson. Clinical and Health Psychology Research Centre, School of Human and Life Sciences, Roehampton University, Whitelands College. 2006.

The necessity of Rostrolateral Prefrontal Cortex for Higher-Level Sequential Behavior. TheresaM., Desrochers ChristopherH. Chatham, David Badre. Neuron. 2015

Auld lang syne: success predictors, change processes, and self-reported outcomes of New Year's resolvers and non-resolvers. Norcross JC, Mrykalo MS, Nlagys MD, J Clin. Psychol. 2002.

A systematic review and meta-analysis of applications of the Self-Report Habit Index to nutrition and physical activity behaviours. Gardner B, de Bruijn GJ, Lally P. Ann Behav Med. 2011

Deep Sleep Helps the Brain Wash Away Toxic Proteins. Maiken Nedergaard, University of Rochester Medical Center (URMC). Science. 2013.

A Daily Diary Study on Sleep Quality and Procrastination at Work: The Moderating Role of Trait Self-Control. Wendelien van Eerde and Merlijn Venus. Amsterdam Business School, University of Amsterdam. Front. Psychol. 2018

ß-Amyloid accumulation in the human brain after one night of sleep deprivation. Ehsan Shokri-Kojori, Gene-Jack Wang, Corinde E. Wiers, Sukru B. Demiral, Min Guo, Sung Won Kim, Elsa Lindgren, Veronica Ramirez, Amna Zehra, Clara Freeman, Gregg Miller, Peter Manza, Tansha Srivastava, Susan De Santi, Dardo Tomasi, Helene Benveniste, and Nora D. Volkow. PNAS. 2018

Circadian topology of metabolism. Bass J (2012). Nature.

Overview of circadian rhythms. Vitaterna MH, Takahashi JS, Turek FW (2001). NIAAA

Mind-altering microorganisms: the impact of the gut microbiota on brain and behaviour. John F. Cryan and Timothy G. Dinan. Laboratory of Neurogastroenterology, Alimentary Pharmabiotic Centre, University College Cork, Cork, Ireland. Department of Anatomy and Neuroscience, University College Cork, Cork, Ireland. Department of Psychiatry, University College Cork, Cork, Ireland. Published online. 2012

Good or bad: gut bacteria in human health and diseases. Hao Wang, Chuan-Xian Wei , Lu Min & Ling-Yun Zhu. Published online. 2018

Printed in Great
Britain
by Amazon

31675141R00087